Fast Facts

Fas┌
L┘

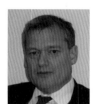

Chris Hatton MA FRCP FRCPath
Consultant Haematologist
Department of Haematology
John Radcliffe Hospital, Oxford, UK

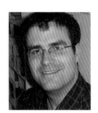

Graham Collins MA MRCP
Lymphoma Research Fellow
Department of Haematology
John Radcliffe Hospital, Oxford, UK

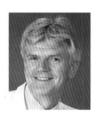

John Sweetenham MD FRCP
Professor and Director of Clinical Research
Taussig Cancer Center, Cleveland Clinic
Cleveland, Ohio, USA

Declaration of Independence
This book is as balanced and as practical as we can make it.
Ideas for improvement are always welcome: feedback@fastfacts.com

HEALTH PRESS

Fast Facts: Lymphoma
First published April 2008
Reprinted 2008

Health Press Limited, Elizabeth House, Queen Street, Abingdon,
Oxford OX14 3LN, UK
Tel: +44 (0)1235 523233
Fax: +44 (0)1235 523238

Book orders can be placed by telephone or via the website.
For regional distributors or to order via the website, please go to:
www.fastfacts.com
For telephone orders, please call +44 (0)1752 202301 (UK and Europe),
1 800 247 6553 (USA, toll free), +1 419 281 1802 (Americas) or +61 (0)2 9351 6173
(Asia–Pacific).

Fast Facts is a trademark of Health Press Limited.

The photographs in Chapter 3 are reproduced courtesy of the Oxford Cytogenetics
Department, Oxford Radcliffe Hospitals Trust, and Professor K Gatter, University of
Oxford, Oxford, UK.

The publisher and the authors have made every effort to insure the accuracy of this
book, but cannot accept responsibility for any errors or omissions.

For all drugs, please consult the product labeling approved in your country for
prescribing information.

Cover image is a hematoxylin–eosin stained section of a lymphoepithelioid lesion in
the mucosa-associated lymphoid tissue (MALT) lymphoma subtype.

A CIP record for this title is available from the British Library.

ISBN: 978-1-903734-99-5

Hatton, C (Chris)
Fast Facts: Lymphoma/
Chris Hatton, Graham Collins, John Sweetenham

Medical illustrations by Dee McLean, London, UK.
Typesetting and page layout by Zed, Oxford, UK.
Printed by Fine Print (Services) Ltd, Oxford, UK.

Text printed with vegetable inks on biodegradable and
recyclable paper manufactured from sustainable forests.

444   001
Low emissions
during production

Low
chlorine

Sustainable
forests

Glossary of abbreviations

ALK: anaplastic lymphoma kinase

ALL: acute lymphoblastic leukemia

ATLL: adult T-cell leukemia/lymphoma

CD4: (cluster of differentiation 4) glycoprotein marker for T-helper cells

CD8: (cluster of differentiation 8) glycoprotein marker for cytotoxic T cells

cHL: classical Hodgkin lymphoma

CLL: chronic lymphocytic (or lymphatic) leukemia

CNS: central nervous system

CSF: cerebrospinal fluid

CT: computed tomography

DLBCL: diffuse large B-cell lymphoma

EBV: Epstein–Barr virus

EDTA: ethylenediamine tetra-acetic acid

FISH: fluorescent in-situ hybridization

FLIPI: Follicular Lymphoma International Prognostic Index

GCB: germinal-center B cell

G-CSF: granulocyte colony-stimulating factor

HAART: highly active antiretroviral therapy

HLA: human leukocyte antigen

HRP: horseradish peroxidase

HRS: Hodgkin/Reed–Sternberg

HTLV-1: human T-cell lymphotropic virus 1

IPI: International Prognostic Index

L&H: lymphocytic and histiocytic

LBL: lymphoblastic lymphoma

LDH: lactate dehydrogenase

LGL: large granular lymphocyte

LPL: lymphoplasmacytoid lymphoma

MALT: mucosa-associated lymphoid tissue

MHC: major histocompatibility complex (protein)

NHL: Non-Hodgkin lymphoma

nLPHL: nodular lymphocyte-predominant Hodgkin lymphoma

PD: progressive disease

PET: positron emission tomography

PR: partial remission

PTLD: post-transplant lymphoproliferative disorder

REAL: Revised European American Lymphoma (classification)

rHuEpo: recombinant human erythropoietin

SD: stable disease

SEER: Surveillance, Epidemiology and End Results

SLL: small lymphocytic lymphoma

SLVL: splenic lymphoma with villous lymphocytosis

SVC: superior vena cava

TCR: T-cell receptor

WHO: World Health Organization

Chemotherapy regimens

ABVD: doxorubicin (adriamycin), bleomycin, vinblastine, dacarbazine

BEACOPP: bleomycin, etoposide, adriamycin (doxorubicin), cyclophosphamide, oncovin (vincristine), procarbazine, prednisone

CHOP: cyclophosphamide, hydroxydaunorubicin (doxorubicin), oncovin (vincristine), prednisolone

CODOX-M: cyclophosphamide, oncovin (vincristine), doxorubicin, methotrexate

CVP: cyclophosphamide, vincristine, prednisolone

EPOCH: etoposide, prednisone, oncovin (vincristine), cyclophosphamide, hydroxydaunorubicin (doxorubicin)

ESHAP: etoposide, steroid (methylprednisolone), high-dose ara-C (cytarabine), platinum (cisplatin)

HyperCVAD-MA: high-dose, fractionated cyclophosphamide, vincristine, adriamycin (doxorubicin), dexamethasone, methotrexate, cytosine arabinoside

IVAC: ifosfamide, etoposide, ara-C (cytarabine)

R-CHOP: rituximab plus cyclophosphamide, hydroxydaunorubicin (doxorubicin), oncovin (vincristine), prednisolone

R-CVP: rituximab plus cyclophosphamide, vincristine, prednisolone

R-DHAP: rituximab plus dexamethasone, high-dose ara-C (cytarabine), platinum (cisplatin)

R-ESHAP: rituximab plus etoposide, steroid (methylprednisolone), high-dose ara-C (cytarabine), platinum (cisplatin)

R-FMD: rituximab plus fludarabine, mitoxantrone, dexamethasone

R-ICE: rituximab plus ifosfamide, carboplatin, etoposide

Introduction

Lymphoma is an interesting and significant disease in a number of respects. It can affect young patients, and, in some cases, may be curable. Certain forms are increasing in incidence and it is now one of the commonest malignancies of the Western world. However, this is not where its significance ends. The developments in basic and applied sciences have been used in the clinical setting nowhere more notably than in the management of patients with hematologic malignancies. The CHOP chemotherapy regimen in the 1970s constituted a major breakthrough in the treatment of non-Hodgkin lymphomas and, indeed, paved the way for the development of the specialty of medical oncology; this in turn heralded the beginning of truly effective chemotherapy. Simultaneously, improved radiotherapy methods defined early stage Hodgkin lymphoma as a curable entity.

It was on this background that, in the 1980s and 1990s, the development of immunophenotyping and molecular diagnostic techniques allowed greater precision in the classification of lymphoproliferative diseases and a still more rational approach to their management. Targeted biological agents such as rituximab exemplify this approach, and the effects in terms of improved overall survival of patients with lymphoma have been dramatic. Staging techniques have similarly advanced from surgical laparotomy to positron emission tomography.

Fast Facts: Lymphoma aims to outline both a historical and up-to-date perspective of the diagnosis and management of Hodgkin and non-Hodgkin lymphomas. Fundamentally, this book should impart a clear understanding of the nature of lymphoma and the principles of its management. It should therefore be of use to training doctors and specialist nurses in the field of hemato-oncology, as well as being of interest to the inquiring patient or carer who wishes to know more about lymphoma.

Epidemiology

Lymphoma is a malignancy of lymphocytes and their progenitors. The term lymphoma encompasses a broad range of lymphoid malignancies, which is reflected in the complexity of the classification systems (see page 140). Consequently, it is difficult to present an all-encompassing overview of the epidemiology of lymphoma. The task is further hindered by weaknesses inherent in the classification systems available. For example, although the current World Health Organization (WHO) and Revised European American Lymphoma (REAL) classification systems are clinically useful, it is likely that some of the broader categories, such as diffuse large B-cell lymphoma, include several distinct entities, each with its own unique epidemiological and etiologic profile. The most accurate epidemiological data come from the Surveillance, Epidemiology and End Results (SEER) Program of the National Cancer Institute in the USA, which has provided most of the data discussed here.

Incidence

The annual incidence of lymphoma in the USA between 1995 and 1999 was 19.1/100 000, making it the fifth most common cancer. The incidence is slightly lower in Western Europe.

Factors affecting incidence

Age. Overall, incidence increases with age. However, children are more susceptible to certain forms of lymphoma (Table 1.1).

TABLE 1.1

Characteristics of lymphomas in children

- Less common than in adults: annual incidence approximately 0.8–1/100 000
- More often high grade (e.g. lymphoblastic lymphoma, Burkitt lymphoma, anaplastic large-cell lymphoma)
- Decreasing mortality

Sex. The incidence is 50% higher in men. However, certain lymphoma subtypes have a predisposition to affect men or women. For example, mantle cell lymphoma particularly affects men (> 70% of cases), whereas primary mediastinal B-cell lymphoma is more common in women.

Ethnicity. The incidence of non-Hodgkin lymphoma (NHL) is 50% higher in white Americans than black Americans.

Geography. It has long been recognized that certain forms of lymphoma have an increased incidence in certain parts of the world (Figure 1.1). This association is particularly striking for endemic Burkitt lymphoma and adult T-cell leukemia/lymphoma; however, similar associations are also well established for other subtypes. Overall, NHL is most common in the USA, Western Europe and Australia (possibly reflecting the age demographics of these populations). However,

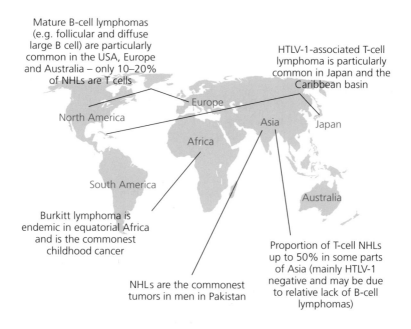

Figure 1.1 Geographical variation of non-Hodgkin lymphoma (NHL) subtypes. HTLV-1, human T-cell lymphotropic virus 1.

Hodgkin lymphoma is considerably more common in the Middle East with incidence rates almost double those of Western Europe.

Changes in incidence. From 1973 to 1990, the annual incidence of NHL in the USA rose by 81% from 10.2 to 18.5/100 000 (Figure 1.2); this increase was observed in all racial groups and in both sexes. This rate of increase has only been surpassed by lung cancer in women and melanoma in both sexes for which specific etiologic factors have been identified (smoking and exposure to ultraviolet radiation, respectively). Recent SEER data suggest, however, that from 1990–1999 the incidence of NHL has plateaued. Interestingly, the incidence of Hodgkin lymphoma has been stable.

Research into the reasons why the incidence of lymphoma has increased so dramatically has so far failed to provide convincing answers. Possible factors that have been identified can be divided into two broad categories:

- relatively uncommon risk factors that carry a high relative risk
- common risk factors that carry a low relative risk.

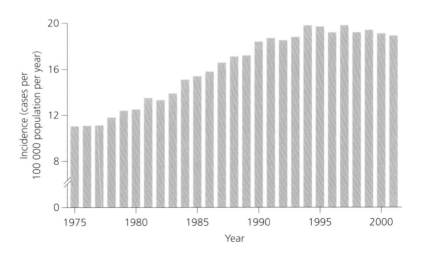

Figure 1.2 Increasing incidence of non-Hodgkin lymphoma in the USA from 1973 to 2001.

Relatively uncommon risk factors with high relative risk.
Immunodeficiency states are the most obvious examples of a relatively
uncommon risk factor that carries a high relative risk. It has been
suggested that the rising incidence of lymphoma reflects an increasing
incidence of immunodeficiency, most obviously due to the emergence
of the human immunodeficiency virus (HIV) and acquired
immunodeficiency syndrome (AIDS). Indeed, HIV/AIDS has been
shown to be a major risk factor for the development of lymphoma,
but it accounts for less than 50% of the increase in incidence seen in
the West. Furthermore, since the advent of highly active antiretroviral
therapy (HAART), the incidence of AIDS-associated lymphoma
has declined.

Common risk factors with low relative risk. Many environmental
factors have been implicated in the development of lymphoma (see
below). Most of these have been identified using case-control
retrospective analyses, which have disadvantages, such as recall
and selection bias, that can reduce the validity of the results. Further
large, prospective, cohort studies are needed, some of which are
ongoing. However, it must be remembered that a relatively innocuous
environmental exposure that carries only a marginally raised relative
risk of developing lymphoma can contribute substantially to a
rising incidence if a sufficiently large number of people are exposed.
Nevertheless, because it is not possible to test for every environmental
exposure that carries only a marginally raised relative risk, it is unlikely
that the rising incidence will ever be fully explained.

Causes of non-Hodgkin lymphoma

Environmental factors

Immunosuppression. There are two relatively common causes
of immunosuppression:

- HIV infection increases the risk of developing NHL more than
  100-fold. The lymphomas are generally aggressive: either diffuse
  large B-cell or Burkitt type (see Chapter 8).
- Patients receiving immunosuppressive drugs following solid organ
  transplantation are at 30–50-fold increased risk of developing NHL;
  Epstein–Barr virus (EBV) is often a cofactor. The drugs impair T-cell

control of EBV-driven polyclonal B-cell activation resulting in polyclonal B-cell proliferation. A dominant B-cell clone can then evolve resulting in lymphoma (see Chapter 8).

Infection (other than HIV) may be an acquired cause of lymphoma (Tables 1.2 and 1.3).

Inflammatory conditions. Certain inflammatory conditions predispose to the development of NHL and particularly extranodal marginal zone/mucosa-associated lymphoid tissue (MALT) lymphomas, which are associated with organ-specific autoimmune conditions. For example, Sjögren syndrome (an autoimmune condition affecting the salivary and lacrimal glands) is associated with a 15-fold increased risk of developing salivary or lacrimal MALT lymphomas, and Hashimoto disease (an autoimmune condition affecting the thyroid gland) predisposes to thyroid MALT lymphoma.

Pesticide exposure. Numerous studies have implicated pesticides and herbicides in the etiology of NHL including organophosphates, phenoxyacetic acid herbicides and triazine herbicides. However, the

TABLE 1.2

Bacteria known to be associated with lymphoma

	Type of lymphoma
Helicobacter pylori	Seropositivity to *H. pylori* increases the risk of gastric mucosa-associated lymphoid tissue (MALT) lymphoma six-fold; treatment with antibiotics to eradicate *H. pylori* leads to regression in most cases of localized disease
Campylobacter jejuni	Immunoproliferative small intestinal disease (α heavy-chain disease), which is mainly seen in the Mediterranean, is associated with *C. jejuni*
Chlamydia psittaci	Reports conflict over the association between ocular adnexal MALT lymphoma, which affects the tissues surrounding the eye, and *C. psittaci*
Borrelia burgdorferi	Primary B-cell lymphoma of the skin is another rare subtype of MALT lymphoma, which is thought to be associated with *B. burgdorferi*

TABLE 1.3

Viruses other than HIV known to be associated with lymphoma

	Type of lymphoma
Human T-cell lymphotropic virus 1 (HTLV-1)	Adult T-cell leukemia/lymphoma (ATLL): common in Japan and the Caribbean basin, some cases also reported in South America; infection with HTLV-1 confers a 1–2% lifetime risk of developing ATLL
Epstein–Barr virus (EBV)	Up to 90% of the population become infected with EBV (Figure 1.3), which is implicated in various types of lymphoma • 50% of cases of Hodgkin lymphoma are positive for EBV in the USA and Western Europe, and the rate is higher in developing countries; a large cohort study has shown that symptomatic EBV infection as a young adult confers a four-fold relative risk of developing EBV-positive Hodgkin lymphoma • EBV is associated with almost 100% of cases of endemic Burkitt lymphoma (malarial infection probably acting as a cofactor) and around 50% of sporadic Burkitt lymphoma • EBV is often a co-factor in post-transplantation lymphoproliferative disease
Hepatitis C virus	Splenic marginal zone lymphoma has been reported to have an association with hepatitis C infection

results are inconsistent with wide variations in the estimates of risk. This is presumably because most investigations have been case-control studies in which the estimation of risk is fraught with difficulty. Some studies have also demonstrated an association between specific pesticides and herbicides and NHL subtypes but, again, the results are inconsistent.

Pesticide exposure is not only relevant to the small proportion of the population who work in agriculture, as studies have convincingly shown that pesticide exposure in the general population is increasing dramatically. Only a small (and therefore difficult to demonstrate) relative risk may account for a significant proportion of lymphoma cases.

Blood transfusion. Increased use of blood transfusions has coincided with the increased incidence of lymphoma. It has been postulated that the immunosuppressive action of a blood transfusion and/or the inherent risk of spreading bloodborne viruses is involved. However, results from cohort and case-control studies are conflicting.

Genetic factors. Only a few inherited conditions predispose to lymphoma development. These conditions are largely primary immunodeficiency states. They are all rare and so do not contribute significantly to the overall prevalence of NHL.

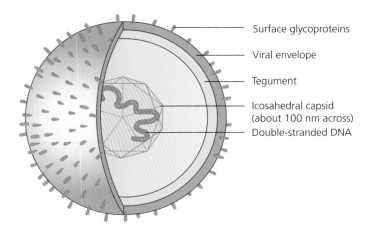

Surface glycoproteins

Viral envelope

Tegument

Icosahedral capsid
(about 100 nm across)

Double-stranded DNA

EBV infects two types of cell
- Epithelial cells, usually of the oropharynx, are thought to be the first cell type infected (primary infection). EBV actively replicates within the cell, causing it to lyse and shed virus, resulting in the familiar sore throat of glandular fever. As the cells lyse, the virus may then spread to B cells
- Memory B cells are often infected. The virus becomes latent, which means that it does not undergo active replication and is hidden from the immune system. At this stage, only a few of the 100 or so viral genes are expressed. A number of latency proteins may act to cause cancer

Figure 1.3 The Epstein–Barr virus (EBV), a member of the herpes virus family.

Examples include:
- Wiskott–Aldrich syndrome
- ataxia–telangiectasia
- X-linked lymphoproliferative syndrome
- common variable immune deficiency.

In each case, a cofactor is needed for lymphoma development, such as EBV.

More subtle defects in immunoregulation are also hypothesized to increase the risk of NHL. A clear clustering of cases is seen in some families but no genetic abnormalities have been found. These may either represent cases of a shared environmental exposure or an as yet undiscovered genetic susceptibility.

Key points – epidemiology

- The epidemiology of lymphoma is difficult to study owing to the existence of so many different subtypes of the disease, each with its own epidemiology and associated causative factors.
- A striking and, as yet, unexplained increase in the incidence of non-Hodgkin lymphoma has been observed over recent years.
- An understanding of the epidemiology has, in some instances, led to an understanding of causative factors such as human T-cell lymphotropic virus infection causing adult T-cell leukemia/lymphoma.
- Various other subtypes of lymphoma have been linked with infection, particularly immunosuppression-related lymphomas caused by Epstein–Barr virus infection and mucosa-associated lymphoid tissue lymphomas caused by various bacterial infections.
- Large cohort studies are required to verify many of the potential causative factors.

Key references

American Society of Hematology. *Education Program Book.* www.asheducationbook.org [Accessed 9 August 2007].

Pagano JS. Viruses and lymphomas. *N Engl J Med* 2002;347:78–9.

Ries LAG, Melbert D, Krapcho M et al., eds. *SEER Cancer Statistics Review 1975–2004.* Bethesda, MD: National Cancer Institute, 2006.

Surveillance Epidemiology and End Results. *SEER Cancer Statistics Review, 1975–2004.* www.seer.cancer.gov/csr/1975_2004/ [Accessed 9 August 2007].

Thorley-Lawson DA, Gross A. Persistence of the Epstein–Barr virus and the origins of associated lymphomas. *N Engl J Med* 2004; 350:1328–37.

Vose JM, Chiu BC, Cheson BD et al. Update on epidemiology and therapeutics for non-Hodgkin's lymphoma. *Hematology Am Soc Hematol Educ Program* 2002: 241–62.

2 Cellular and molecular aspects

The purpose of the immune system is to fight infection. Cells and molecules of the immune system have evolved to recognize components of microorganisms as 'foreign' or 'non-self'. These 'non-self' components are molecular fragments called antigens.

The immune system can be divided in two, conceptually. The innate immune system is a complex network of cells and molecules that do not have the property of 'memory'. In other words, the innate immune system's response to an antigen will be broadly the same, irrespective of any previous encounter. Conversely, the adaptive immune system has 'memory'. Therefore, an encounter with an antigen will strengthen any subsequent responses.

The main cellular mediators of adaptive immunity are lymphocytes. There are two types of lymphocyte: the B lymphocyte (or B cell) and the T lymphocyte (or T cell). Each type of lymphocyte makes a receptor that can recognize and respond to a specific antigen. The B-cell antigen receptor is called immunoglobulin which, when secreted in its soluble form, is called antibody and is composed of two heavy and two light chains (Figure 2.1). There are various classes of immunoglobulin (IgG, IgA, IgM, IgD and IgE) that determine the effector functions of the antibody. For example, IgE is able to bind to a type of cell called the mast cell and cause the release of histamine, whereas IgA is particularly adapted for secretion, which enables it to act at the lining of the airways or gut. IgM and IgD are produced by B cells before they have encountered antigen, whereas after antigen exposure, the immunoglobulin can switch to any of the classes mentioned above. The T-cell antigen receptor is simply called the T-cell receptor (TCR) and is composed of two chains (α and β or γ and δ; Figure 2.2).

Lymphomas arise from a single abnormal lymphocyte. Genetic changes within the lymphocyte lead to an accumulation of cells, every one of which has arisen from a single cell (a clonal population). Different types of lymphoma are thought to exist because genetic

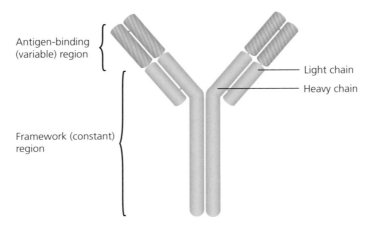

Figure 2.1 Immunoglobulin (antibody) molecule.

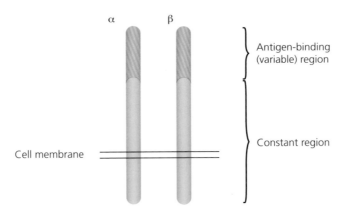

Figure 2.2 T-cell receptor.

changes occur in lymphocytes at different stages of their life cycle. Therefore, to understand lymphoma classification it is important to have some knowledge of the life cycle of B and T lymphocytes.

Lymphocyte life cycle

Both B and T lymphocytes arise from a common lymphoid progenitor cell in the bone marrow.

B-cell development occurs in two stages:
- antigen-independent
- antigen-dependent.

Antigen-independent development takes place predominantly in the bone marrow, which is one of two primary lymphoid organs. The earliest recognizable cell in the B-cell lineage is called the pro-B cell. This matures to produce the pre-B cell, which expresses immunoglobulin internally within the cytoplasm (along with a receptor on the surface called the pre-B cell receptor). This in turn develops into the immature B cell, which expresses intact immunoglobulin (IgM or IgD) on the surface of the cell. The main molecular event during the antigen-independent phase is rearrangement of the heavy- and light-chain genes that code for the immunoglobulin receptor, thereby generating a vast range of B-cell receptors capable of recognizing large numbers of new antigens.

At this stage, if the immunoglobulin receptor on the surface of the B cell encounters an antigen it recognizes as 'self' or 'host', such as a protein on a neighboring cell, the lymphocyte either dies by apoptosis or, more commonly, undergoes a process called receptor editing which results in an immunoglobulin molecule of different affinity from the original one. This prevents the B cells from eliciting immune responses against the host in the future. The surviving B cells are then transported in the bloodstream to the spleen where they undergo further development (in the form of cells called transitional B cells) to result in mature (although still antigen naive) B cells.

There are two forms of mature B cell: the follicular B cell and the marginal zone B cell. Marginal zone B cells only exist in the spleen and can respond very rapidly to bloodborne antigens, producing an IgM antibody response. Follicular B cells may stay in the spleen or be transported to other secondary lymphoid organs, such as a lymph node or Peyer's patch (located in the lining of the gut) where they undergo antigen-dependent development.

Antigen-dependent development takes place in the secondary lymphoid organs, which are the sites of interaction between the adaptive immune system and invading microorganisms. The structure within the lymphoid organs in which this interaction occurs is called the germinal center. Within the germinal center, specialized cells called follicular dendritic cells present the invading microorganisms' foreign antigen to B cells (Figure 2.3); if the B cells recognize the foreign antigen they are rescued from cell death by the intervention of T cells, allowing a population of B cells to survive that are capable of recognizing foreign organisms and producing antibodies that attack them. Two molecular events take place during this phase.

- Somatic hypermutation introduces mutations into regions of the immunoglobulin genes. This refines or hones the antigen specificity of the immunoglobulin molecule and enables the immune system to counter foreign organisms more efficiently. Mutations that result in a lower affinity immunoglobulin molecule lead to death of the cell by apoptosis.
- Class switch recombination switches the class of immunoglobulin expressed by the cell, thereby changing the effector functions the antibody is capable of mediating. It therefore broadens the ability of the immune system to destroy the invader.

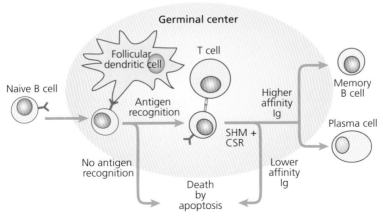

Figure 2.3 Antigen-dependent B-cell development. CSR, class switch recombination; Ig, immunoglobulin; SHM, somatic hypermutation.

For most B cells that enter the germinal center, the end result is death by apoptosis. However, for those cells that have a high affinity immunoglobulin for the antigen being encountered, the B cell can become either a memory B cell (which enables the body to recognize the same microorganism more quickly on subsequent exposures) or an antibody-producing plasma cell. The plasma cells are short lived, unless they leave the environment of the lymph node and hone to a niche within the bone marrow in which they can survive for a considerable length of time.

T-cell maturation occurs in the other primary lymphoid organ, the thymus. The formation of a TCR is analogous to that of an immunoglobulin molecule in a B cell. The four TCR genes (α, β, γ and δ) undergo rearrangement in a similar way to the heavy- and light-chain immunoglobulin genes. The result is the expression of a TCR consisting of either α and β or γ and δ chains each with a defined antigen specificity.

Mature T cells can be broadly classified into two types: T-helper cells (which are primarily involved in coordinating the immune response to a given invader) and cytotoxic T cells (which, as their name suggests, can kill cells infected with microorganisms). The two cell types can be recognized by the presence of a specific molecule on their cell surface: helper T cells express CD4 whereas cytotoxic T cells express CD8. T-cell maturation occurs in four main phases (Figure 2.4).

- β (or δ) chain expression is the first step. At this point the cell expresses neither CD4 nor CD8 (a so-called double-negative cell).
- α and β (or γ and δ) chain expression then occurs, at which point the cell expresses both CD4 and CD8 (a double-positive cell).
- Positive selection is the next step and is the process whereby T cells with TCRs that bind antigen expressed in combination with a protein called the major histocompatibility complex (MHC) on the surface of thymic epithelial cells are rescued from apoptosis. This enables the T cells to respond to antigen presented by the host.
- Negative selection is the final process whereby T cells with TCRs that react strongly with antigen expressed in combination with MHC by dendritic cells are made to die by apoptosis. This helps prevent T cells from entering the circulation and then attacking the host's own body.

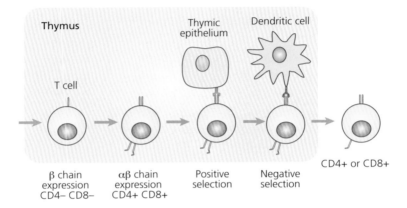

Thymus

T cell

Thymic
epithelium

Dendritic cell

CD4+ or CD8+

β chain	αβ chain	Positive	Negative
expression	expression	selection	selection
CD4– CD8–	CD4+ CD8+		

Figure 2.4 T-cell maturation in the thymus.

The end result is a mature, single positive (either CD4 or CD8 positive) T cell.

Normal lymph-node architecture

Due to the genetic insults occurring in the lymph node, namely somatic hypermutation and class switch recombination, many lymphomas arise within this structure. The normal lymph node is encased by a capsule, below which is the subcapsular sinus through which lymphocytes enter the lymph node. Deep to the sinus lies the cortex of the lymph node, which contains the primary and secondary follicles (Figure 2.5).

- The primary follicles are composed of resting B cells.
- The secondary follicles appear when antigen is encountered and are characterized by the presence of germinal centers, which are where antigen is presented to B cells by follicular dendritic cells; the B cells then either proliferate or die by apoptosis depending on the affinity of their immunoglobulin receptor for the antigen (see page 21). Secondary follicles also have a mantle zone composed of resting B cells that have not yet encountered antigen.

Alongside the cortex lies the paracortex, which is predominantly composed of T cells. Deep to the cortex and paracortex lies the medulla of the lymph node. This contains medullary cords (composed mainly of

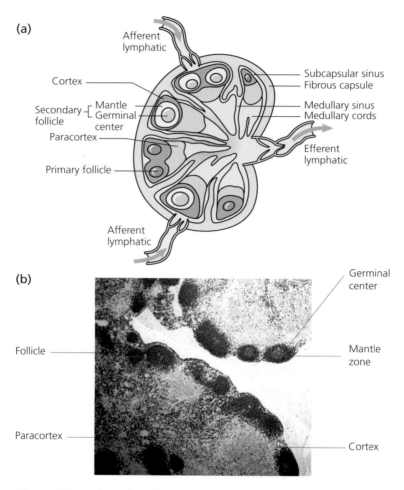

Figure 2.5 Lymph-node architecture. (a) Structure of a normal lymph node. (b) Normal lymph node stained with anti-CD20 antibody highlighting the B-cell areas.

plasma cells and macrophages) and the medullary sinus, through which lymphocytes and fluid pass when exiting the node.

Origin of specific lymphoid disorders

It has been suggested that different types of lymphoma arise because cancer-causing insults occur in lymphocytes at different stages of their life cycle. A combination of basic morphology, flow cytometry and immunohistochemistry (see page 29) has been used to support this concept. The most basic distinction is whether a B-cell lymphoma is derived from cells before or after they have traversed the germinal center (Table 2.1). This is relatively straightforward to discover because, if they have entered the antigen-dependent part of the life cycle and are within (or have been through) the germinal center, the immunoglobulin genes will have undergone somatic hypermutation. This can be determined using specialized molecular testing. In addition, certain cell surface markers indicate a germinal center origin.

Molecular basis of cancer

Any cancer can be considered as a process characterized by unregulated cell division, cell growth and impaired cellular maturation. These processes are normally carefully controlled by a complex interplay of

TABLE 2.1

Proposed classification of B-cell lymphoid disorders based on life cycle

Pre-germinal center
- Lymphoblastic lymphoma/acute lymphoblastic leukemia
- Some subtypes of small lymphocytic lymphoma
- Mantle cell lymphoma

Germinal-center derived
- Follicular lymphoma
- Burkitt lymphoma
- Some types of diffuse large B-cell lymphoma

Post-germinal center
- Lymphoplasmacytoid lymphoma
- Some subtypes of small lymphocytic lymphoma
- Hodgkin lymphoma
- Some types of diffuse large B-cell lymphoma

genes and their protein products but, because of damage to the genetic structure, are fundamentally disturbed in a cancer cell. Cancer can, therefore, be considered a genetic disease. This does not mean it is hereditary, but rather is due to the accumulation of a number of acquired genetic changes that cause the transformation of a normal cell into a malignant cell. The genetic changes result in either over- or underexpression of the genes involved. There are two main classes of gene involved: oncogenes and tumor suppressor genes (Table 2.2).

Oncogenes are overexpressed in the process of malignant transformation. Usually only one copy of the gene needs to be affected for expression of a malignant phenotype. The unmutated form of an oncogene found in normal cells is called a proto-oncogene.

Tumor suppressor genes. When these genes are functioning, they prevent malignant transformation. Underexpression through inactivation of both copies of the gene is therefore usually required for malignant transformation to occur. The two copies of the tumor suppressor gene may be inactivated by different processes. For example,

TABLE 2.2

Examples of oncogenes and tumor suppressor genes

	Function of protein
Oncogenes	
Ras	Involved in cell growth and proliferation
Cyclin D1	Involved in driving the cell cycle forward
c-myc	Involved in regulating the balance between cell growth and apoptosis
Bcl2	Inhibits apoptosis
Tumor suppressor genes	
Retinoblastoma gene	Slows down progression through the cell cycle
p53	Halts the cell cycle in response to DNA damage

a deletion process may affect one copy, whereas a point mutation may affect the other. The end result must be silencing of the expression of both copies before malignant transformation is possible.

Molecular mechanisms altering gene function in lymphomas

Various molecular mechanisms are responsible for the alteration of gene expression seen in malignant transformation.

Deletion of chromosomal material. For example, in non-Hodgkin lymphomas, deletion of part of the short arm of chromosome 8 is a well-described phenomenon. It is thought that this leads to loss of a critical gene that would normally result in the death of the cancerous lymphocyte.

Chromosomal translocations. In numerous lymphoid disorders, a commonly occurring translocation is one that brings an oncogene into proximity with the immunoglobulin heavy-chain gene (*IgH*) on chromosome 14. This places the oncogene under transcriptional control of the immunoglobulin enhancer, which is very active in B lymphocytes, and results in overexpression of the oncogene. The *IgH* gene is the partner in a number of different translocations associated with a number of different lymphomas, such as: t(14;18) in follicular lymphoma; t(11;14) in mantle cell lymphoma; and t(8;14) in Burkitt lymphoma. Rearrangement of the *IgH* gene is a normal occurrence in B-cell development and it is thought that this propensity to recombine may be the reason it is so relatively frequently involved in malignant translocations.

A point mutation, such as a premature stop codon, may be introduced that results in a short, non-functioning protein product; alternatively, a different amino acid residue may be inserted that could affect protein function, causing constitutive activation or inactivation.

Methylation of cytosine residues in the promoter sites of genes silences expression of that gene, resulting in an alteration of gene function with no change in the genetic sequence itself. A number of potential tumor suppressors have been identified that can be silenced by methylation. The SHP-1 promoter is methylated in T-cell

27

lymphomas. This silencing of a suppressor gene results in upregulation of cell signaling and subsequent uncontrolled activation of the cell cycle.

Uniparental disomy is when both copies of a whole, or part of, a chromosome are of paternal or maternal origin. In cancer, this may occur as an acquired phenomenon, thought to be due to an abnormality during cell division. This means that if one copy of a tumor suppressor gene was mutated on the paternal copy of the chromosome, then acquired uniparental disomy can replace the normal maternal copy with the abnormal paternal copy. This will then promote cancer formation in the affected cell. Acquired uniparental disomy has recently been reported as a secondary genetic event in mantle cell lymphoma.

Key points – cellular and molecular aspects

- Lymphomas are cancers of lymphocytes, the major cellular components of the adaptive immune response.
- Lymphocytes are formed in an antigen-independent stage in the bone marrow (and thymus for T cells) but need an encounter with antigen in secondary lymphoid tissue to develop further.
- The different types of lymphoma probably arise from different stages of the lymphocyte life cycle.
- Lymphomas arise because of several complex genetic changes involving activation of oncogenes or inactivation of tumor suppressor genes.

Key references

Delves PJ, Martin S, Burton D et al. *Roitt's Essential Immunology.* 11th edn. Ames: Blackwell Publishing, 2006.

Knowles M, Selby P, eds. *Introduction to the Cellular and Molecular Biology of Cancer.* 4th edn. New York: Oxford University Press, 2005.

Kuppers R, Klein U et al. Cellular origin of human B-cell lymphomas. *N Engl J Med* 1999;341:1520–9.

Accurate diagnosis is essential in order to successfully treat any disease. This is a major issue in the case of lymphoma due to the existence of so many different subtypes, many of which respond differently to a given treatment modality. Recent advances in cellular and molecular techniques have revolutionized our understanding of lymphoma as a disease and have paved the way for improved diagnosis and treatment.

Flow cytometry and immunophenotyping

Flow cytometry and immunophenotyping can be used to establish the following characteristics of any particle or cell:

- size
- complexity (for a cell this means its granularity)
- surface characteristics (for a cell this means the proteins expressed on the cell surface).

A flow cytometer is capable of analyzing cells one at a time provided the cells are in a fluid phase. Flow cytometry is therefore ideally suited to the analysis of blood samples. However, the technique is also increasingly used to analyze diseased lymph nodes, though the tissue must first be disrupted. Each blood or lymph-node cell scatters a beam of light from a laser in two different ways (Figure 3.1): the forward scattering reflects the size of the cell and the sideways scattering reflects the granularity of the cell. Lymphocytes are small, agranular cells and therefore tend to exhibit a low forward and sideways light scattering.

To determine the proteins expressed on the cell surface, the cells are first mixed with an antibody specific to the protein (antigen) in question. This antibody is linked to a fluorescent marker, which will emit light if it is bound to the cell when it passes through the flow cytometer. The strength of the emitted light is measured by a detector, which then provides information about the relative amount of antigen expressed on the cell surface. More than one protein can be assessed at the same time, as each antibody being used can be linked to markers that emit light of different frequencies. The process of using antibodies to

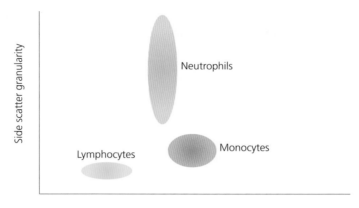

Figure 3.1 Normal forward and side scattering of light by white blood cells, measured by a flow cytometer. The greater the forward scatter, the bigger the cell and the greater the side scatter, the more granular the cell.

define the phenotype of a cell is called immunophenotyping. The immunophenotypes of normal mature T cells and B cells are listed in Table 3.1.

Immunophenotyping is invaluable in the diagnosis of lymphoid disorders. It can help determine:

• clonality
• disease subtype.

Clonality. In B-cell lymphoproliferative disorders, clonality is demonstrated when all of the lymphocytes express either κ or λ light chains. No such test is available to demonstrate the clonality of T cells; clonality is shown by molecular tests that demonstrate a single pattern of rearrangement of the genes of the TCR.

Disease subtype. Certain subtypes of lymphoproliferative disorders are associated with specific patterns of cell surface protein expression, which can be detected by immunophenotyping. In many instances, the pattern is thought to reflect the stage of lymphocyte development at which the malignant change occurred (Table 3.2).

TABLE 3.1

Typical immunophenotypes of B cells and T cells

B cell	T cell
• CD19	• CD3
• CD20	• CD5
• CD79a	• CD7
• CD 79b	• CD4 or CD8 (normal ratio 3:2)
• κ or λ (normal ratio 3:2)	• αβ TCR or γδ TCR

TCR, T-cell receptor.

TABLE 3.2

Typical immunophenotypes associated with class of lymphoproliferative disorder

Mantle cell lymphoma	Follicular lymphoma	Adult T-cell leukemia/lymphoma
CD5	CD10	CD2
CD19	CD19	CD3
CD20 (bright)	CD20	CD4
CD79b	CD79a&b	CD5
FMC7	FMC7	CD7-
SmIg (moderate)	SmIg (bright)	CD25

SmIg, surface membrane immunoglobulin.

Basic histology

The histological appearance of a tissue section obtained at biopsy is essential for lymphoma diagnosis. Much information can be gained from a simple hematoxylin–eosin stain. For example, identification of the typical Hodgkin/Reed–Sternberg cell leads to a diagnosis of classical Hodgkin lymphoma (Figure 3.2), while replacement of the normal lymph-node architecture by monotypic

31

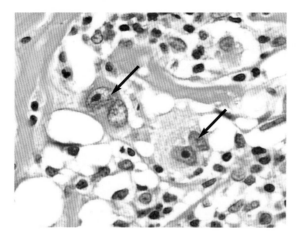

Figure 3.2
Hematoxylin–eosin stain showing two typical Hodgkin/ Reed–Sternberg cells (arrowed) of classical Hodgkin lymphoma.

lymphocytes in follicles points to a diagnosis of follicular lymphoma (Figure 3.3).

Immunohistochemistry

Immunohistochemistry is based on a similar principle to that of immunophenotyping using the flow cytometer. The main difference is that immunohistochemistry uses a fixed tissue section. An antibody targeted against the protein of interest and linked to an enzyme, usually horseradish peroxidase (HRP), is incubated with the tissue section. Unbound antibody is then washed off and a dye is added that turns brown in the presence of HRP. Cells expressing the protein of interest will therefore stain brown (Figure 3.4).

Cytogenetics

Cytogenetics is the study of chromosomes. In hematologic disorders, including lymphomas, abnormalities in both the number and structure of chromosomes are associated with malignant cells. Identification of these abnormalities using various cytogenetic techniques can aid diagnosis.

Karyotyping is conducted on cells in the metaphase (i.e. the stage in the cell cycle when the cell is about to divide). Cells for analysis are obtained from a blood sample, or a bone-marrow or lymph-node

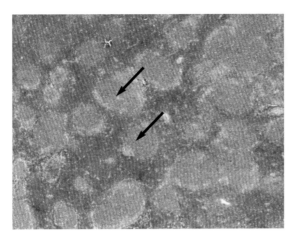

Figure 3.3
Hematoxylin–eosin stain showing typical follicular architecture in follicular lymphoma (neoplastic follicles arrowed).

Figure 3.4 CD10+ lymphocytes in follicular lymphoma.

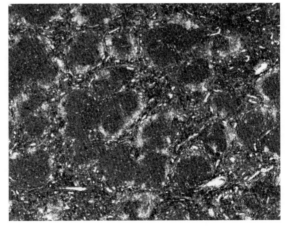

biopsy. The cells are stimulated to grow using a chemical called a mitogen, and a drug is then added that prevents the completion of mitosis, therefore enhancing the yield of cells in metaphase. The nucleus of the cell is made to swell enabling a more detailed look at the chromosomes.

To aid interpretation of any cytogenetic changes, the chromosomes are exposed to trypsin and then stained using Giemsa. This results in alternating light and dark bands, so-called G-banding (Figure 3.5). Each chromosome has a distinct banding pattern enabling identification. Abnormal karyotypes are often found in lymphoid disorders.

33

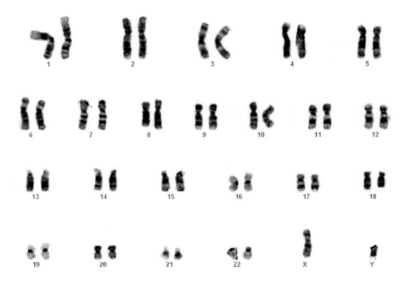

Figure 3.5 Normal human male karyogram stained by a G-banding method.

The most important cytogenetic changes are:
- translocations
- deletions
- aneuploidy
- inversions.

Translocations. A reciprocal translocation occurs when there is an exchange of chromosomal material between two different pairs (non-homologous) of chromosomes. After the translocation, the chromosome is referred to as the derivative chromosome (Figure 3.6). An example is Burkitt lymphoma, which is associated in most cases with a reciprocal translocation between chromosomes 8 and 14.

Deletions of chromosomal material are frequently seen in lymphoid disorders. However, such changes are usually non-specific. An example is del(17p), which is found in a large number of different types of non-Hodgkin lymphoma.

Aneuploidy means that there are more or fewer chromosomes than the normal diploid number. An aggressive form of mantle cell lymphoma (the blastoid variant) is well known to harbor chromosomes in the tetraploid (four copies) range.

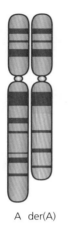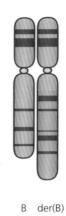

Figure 3.6 Schematic diagram of a balanced, reciprocal translocation.

A der(A)   B   der(B)

Inversions occur when a piece of chromosomal material inverts with respect to its chromosome of origin. For example, certain forms of T-cell proliferation are associated with inversion of part of chromosome 14.

Fluorescent in-situ hybridization

Fluorescent in-situ hybridization (FISH) is used to identify chromosomal abnormalities that are difficult to recognize by conventional cytogenetics (Figure 3.7) and can be performed on either interphase or metaphase cells.

The technique is generally faster than conventional cytogenetics, so can be used to obtain rapid results. This is particularly so for interphase FISH, which does not require cell growth. However, because the chromosomes are more condensed, the interphase FISH results are often harder to read. An example in mantle cell lymphoma is shown in Figure 3.8.

The FISH process is as follows.

- The sample DNA (either metaphase chromosomes or interphase nuclei) is first denatured by heating. This separates the double strands of the DNA helix.

- DNA probes are then added. These are complementary to the DNA being analyzed and contain incorporated fluorescent nucleotides.

35

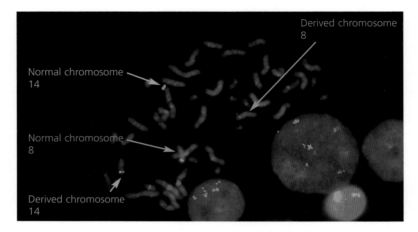

Figure 3.7 Metaphase fluorescent in-situ hybridization showing t(8;14) in Burkitt lymphoma. The translocation is marked by the coming together of the red and green fluorescent probes.

- As the DNA reanneals (reforms double strands), the probes hybridize to the DNA.
- A fluorescence microscope can then be used to detect hybridization of the probes to the DNA.

The disadvantage of FISH is that in order to use the appropriate probes the clinician does need to have an idea of which cytogenetic abnormality to look for.

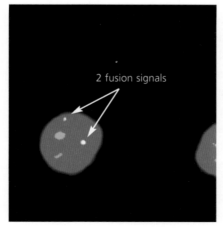

Figure 3.8 Interphase fluorescent in-situ hybridization in a case of mantle cell lymphoma, showing a translocation involving chromosomes 11 and 14. These probes are also fusion probes, the abnormal signal being a fusion of red and green to give a pale yellow color.

Molecular genetic techniques

Polymerase chain reaction (PCR) is a technique that enables very small amounts of DNA (or RNA) to be amplified and detected. Although not widely used in routine clinical laboratories, PCR may be used in the future to identify very small amounts of lymphoma-associated genetic changes (such as translocations) that cannot be detected by cytogenetics or FISH. Detection of so-called minimal residual disease may then dictate further treatment and reduce relapse rates.

Gene-expression microarrays. An important molecular genetic technique that may affect the diagnosis and prognosis of lymphoma is gene-expression microarray technology. There are approximately 20 000 genes in the human genome, and it has been appreciated for some time that in any given malignant condition there are likely to be many genes whose expression is either up- or down-regulated. Microarray technology enables the global analysis of changes in gene expression. It was hypothesized that the patterns of up- and down-regulation detected by gene expression microarrays may be useful in determining new subtypes of lymphoma that have prognostic importance and may, therefore, affect treatment decisions.

In lymphoma, the major impact so far has been in subtyping cases of diffuse large B-cell lymphoma (DLBCL). This group of lymphoma is likely to represent several different entities with distinct epidemiological and etiologic factors. They may also confer a different prognosis to the patient and may be maximally sensitive to different forms of treatment. Expression microarray studies have identified two major groups of DLBCL, which are associated with different outcomes. The first group has a gene expression signature that suggests that the cells have originated from a germinal-center B cell (see page 21). This group is therefore called germinal-center B-cell like and has a relatively good 5-year survival. The second group is rather more heterogenous and is often termed the non-germinal-center B-cell (non-GCB) type. This has a significantly worse 5-year survival rate. It must be said, however, that with the advent of new treatments the differences in outcome between the groups may not be so evident. In particular, the use of rituximab seems to bring the prognosis of the two groups closer together.

More recently, gene-expression microarrays have been applied to the diagnosis of Burkitt lymphoma. Although usually fairly straightforward, the distinction between Burkitt lymphoma and DLBCL can be difficult. A correct diagnosis is very important, however, as the chemotherapy regimens used to treat the two disorders differ greatly.

Studies have shown that gene expression profiling of cases of classic Burkitt lymphoma, diagnosed by expert hematopathologists, identifies a signature which differs from that of DLBCL. What is more interesting is the suggestion of some reports that the microarrays may do better than the expert hematopathologists. Specifically, up to one-third of cases with a Burkitt gene expression profile had been called DLBCL by the pathologist. Conversely, a few cases that were diagnosed as Burkitt lymphoma had the gene expression profile of DLBCL. However, the issue is still far from clear. For example, it is unclear whether the groups identified by microarray technology are more clinically homogenous than similar groups identified by the pathologist. It is also unclear whether the outcome for the groups would be better if diagnosed on the basis of microarrays as opposed to by pathologists. It must also be remembered that the process of gene-expression microarray is laborious and expensive. There are also issues over the reproducibility of results, particularly when the procedure is performed by different laboratories. Microarray technology is therefore a long way from being used routinely either to aid diagnosis or to provide prognostic information.

Tissue microarrays. The problems associated with expression microarrays prompted histopathologists to develop a technique involving multiple small samples of the same tissue placed on a microscope slide. This permits immunohistochemistry on each separate sample, so that a high number of antigens can be analyzed. The hope is that the key antigens discovered by the use of expression microarrays can then be analyzed routinely in the diagnostic laboratory with tissue microarrays. However, when this technique has been applied to detecting subtypes of DLBCL, results from tissue microarrays do not always correlate with the expression microarray data. Thus, this technique, too, is some distance from being used routinely in the management of patients with lymphoma.

Key points – diagnostic laboratory techniques

- New molecular and cellular techniques have revolutionized the diagnosis of lymphoma.
- Immunophenotyping and immunohistochemistry analyze the expression of proteins on the cell surface (or sometimes within the cytoplasm or nucleus).
- Karyotyping and fluorescent in-situ hybridization analysis reveal the chromosomal changes in the cell.
- Gene-expression microarray profiling has led to subtyping cases of diffuse large B-cell lymphomas and may improve the diagnosis of Burkitt lymphoma.
- An increased understanding of the molecular and cellular basis of lymphomas may lead to improved targeting of treatment.

Key references

Atlas of Genetics and Cytogenetics in Oncology and Haematology http://atlasgeneticsoncology.org [Accessed 30 January 2008]

Harris NL, Horning SJ. Burkitt's lymphoma – the message from microarrays. *N Engl J Med* 2006;354:2495–8.

Knowles M, Selby P, eds. *Introduction to the Cellular and Molecular Biology of Cancer.* 4th edn. New York: Oxford University Press, 2005.

Kuppers R, Klein U, Hansmann ML et al. Cellular origin of human B-cell lymphomas. *N Engl J Med* 1999;341:1520–9.

Rosenwald A, Wright G et al. The use of molecular profiling to predict survival after chemotherapy for diffuse large-B-cell lymphoma. *N Engl J Med* 2002;346:1937–47.

This chapter offers a broad outline of the complex subjects of diagnosis, staging and treatment of a patient with lymphoma; the individual lymphoma entities and treatment modalities will be discussed in more detail in subsequent chapters. In particular, see Chapters 5–9 for a more detailed discussion of the individual lymphoma entities, Chapter 10 for detail on treatment modalities and Chapter 11 on management of side effects of the treatments. Chapter 3 covers laboratory diagnostic techniques.

To understand the management principles of lymphoma it is necessary to understand its biology and natural history. Three important statements can be made about lymphomas.

- Lymphomas are the fifth most common malignancy in the USA.
- Although the most common age of presentation of lymphoma is 60–70 years, certain subtypes commonly affect young patients (10% of patients with Hodgkin lymphoma are under 16 years old).
- A significant number of lymphomas are curable.

The last point emphasizes the need to optimize the management of these disorders.

The complexity of lymphomas, particularly their pathology, means that all cases should be referred to an expert lymphoma service to ensure that all patients get a considered opinion from a team, which should include radiation oncologists, hemato-oncologists, specialist nurses, radiologists and hematopathologists.

Nodal and extranodal lymphoma

Lymphomas can affect any organ of the body and are divided into:

- nodal lymphomas, affecting the lymph nodes or spleen
- primary extranodal lymphomas, predominantly affecting any other site (e.g. gastrointestinal tract, lung, brain, skin or kidneys; Figure 4.1).

Recognizing that lymphomas may affect sites outside the lymph nodes is important, because it has a direct bearing on their management.

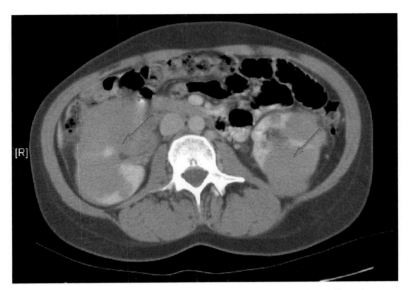

Figure 4.1 Computed tomography scan showing extranodal diffuse large B-cell lymphoma involving both kidneys (a primary extranodal lymphoma; arrowed).

Extranodal sites must be monitored during and after treatment to assess response to therapy. Involvement of two or more extranodal sites confers a worse prognosis and is reflected by an increase in the International Prognostic Index (see page 57 and pages 72–3). Hodgkin lymphoma is almost always nodal, whereas 40% of non-Hodgkin lymphomas (NHLs) involve extranodal sites.

Clinical presentation

Lymphomas are great mimics of other disorders. A lymphoma may present in one of two principal ways:

- mass effect
- systemic effect.

Mass effect. Most lymphomas present as a simple lump – an enlarged lymph node, usually within a nodal group such as the neck or the axilla or groin, but other lymphomas may present as an urgent problem involving critical organs.

Examples of problems caused by enlarged lymph nodes include:
- obstructive jaundice caused by involvement of the lymph nodes adjacent to the porta hepatis (where the bile duct exits the liver)
- renal outflow obstruction or vena caval obstruction caused by rapid and massive involvement of the para-aortic lymph nodes
- superior vena caval obstruction, stridor or dysphagia (Figure 4.2) caused by massive enlargement of mediastinal lymph nodes
- cauda equina or spinal cord compression caused by invasion or compression of the epidural space.

Systemic effect. Lymphoma may present with systemic symptoms such as fever, night sweats and weight loss, and it is always a serious consideration in a patient with a fever of unknown origin. Pruritus is often a presenting complaint. T-cell lymphomas are notorious for producing systemic symptoms with fairly minimal lymphadenopathy, which is probably due to the high levels of cytokine release associated with these types of tumor.

The presentation can be quite variable, because lymphoma may affect any organ of the body. A lymphoma that affects the stomach or bowel

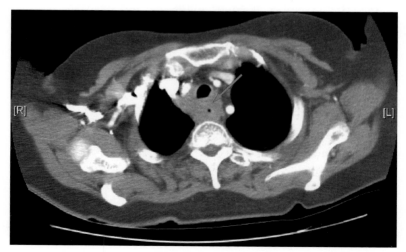

Figure 4.2 Diffuse large B-cell lymphoma affecting the upper mediastinum causing severe dysphagia due to local mass effect. Note the pinpoint esophagus (arrow).

may present as abdominal pain, perforation, bleeding or obstruction. However, a lymphoma that heavily infiltrates the bone marrow may lead to a life-threatening pancytopenia (reduction in circulating blood cells). Occasionally, lymphomas will give rise to autoimmune phenomena, such as hemolysis or peripheral neuropathy.

Management steps

The management of any patient with lymphoma follows the same path:

- biopsy
- staging
- initial therapy
- restaging to determine response to chemotherapy
- completion of therapy.

This principle is just as true at relapse as it is at first presentation.

Biopsy

The surgical removal or biopsy of an enlarged lymph node will provide tissue for diagnosis. Increasingly, guided core biopsy of a lymph-node mass visualized by computed tomography (CT) or another imaging modality is being used to obtain tissue from anatomic sites that are otherwise inaccessible (Figure 4.3). Although this will usually provide adequate tissue for accurate diagnosis using current techniques, excisional biopsy of accessible lymph nodes is preferred.

Pathology. The identification of the specific lymphoma type is complex. Once tissue has been obtained, it is fixed, sectioned and stained with labeled antibodies that identify particular antigens expressed on abnormal cells (see page 29). Almost all lymphomas express the leukocyte common antigen CD45, which defines the tumor as being of hemopoietic origin. Further immunophenotyping will establish whether the tumor is lymphoid or myeloid in origin.

Lymphomas are classified as either Hodgkin lymphoma or NHL and then further subdivided into distinct entities based on the characteristic morphology, immunophenotype and cytogenetic and molecular abnormalities (Figure 4.4). For example, Burkitt, mantle cell and follicular lymphoma have characteristic cytogenetic abnormalities.

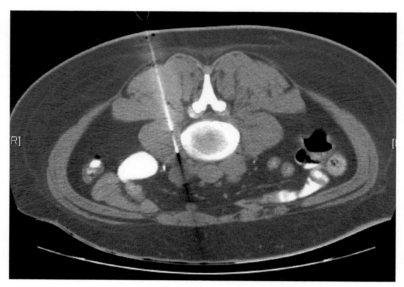

Figure 4.3 Biopsy of retroperitoneal lymphadenopathy guided by computed tomography.

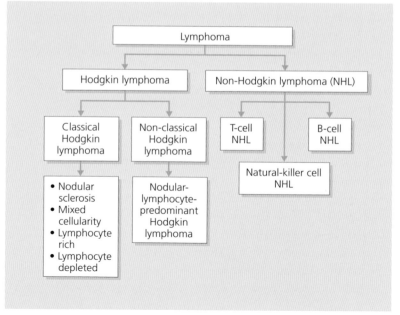

Figure 4.4 Classification of lymphoma.

Tables outlining the complete classification of both Hodgkin lymphoma and NHL are provided on pages 140–2).

Hodgkin lymphoma versus non-Hodgkin lymphoma. The pathological distinction between Hodgkin lymphoma and NHL is usually relatively straightforward, based on histology and immunophenotyping. Most cases of Hodgkin lymphoma, known as classical Hodgkin lymphoma, are characterized by the presence of Hodgkin/Reed–Sternberg (HRS) cells in an appropriate cellular background of infiltrating inflammatory cells. However, one subtype of Hodgkin lymphoma, known as nodular lymphocyte-predominant Hodgkin lymphoma, does not have HRS cells but another characteristic cell known as a lymphocytic and histiocytic (L&H) or 'popcorn' cell (see pages 106–7). Hodgkin lymphoma is a disorder of younger patients, usually spreads contiguously from lymph node to adjacent lymph node and most commonly affects the neck and mediastinum. NHLs tend to affect older patients, are frequently disseminated at first presentation and generally respond less well to treatment. The distinction between these two main types of lymphoma is important, not only because the treatment regimen is different, but also because Hodgkin lymphoma affects young patients, which alters the emphasis when considering the long-term toxicity of the proposed treatment.

Staging

Staging determines the site (Figure 4.5) and extent of a lymphoma. Staging and a general work-up are mandatory in all cases and should include the following investigations.

CT scan or magnetic resonance imaging (MRI) of the chest, abdomen and pelvis should be performed. Positron emission tomography (PET) is currently being evaluated for staging as it may be more sensitive.

Bone-marrow biopsy should be obtained, though it may be omitted in certain lymphoma types.

Blood tests should include blood count, erythrocyte sedimentation rate and biochemical profile to include renal function, liver function and calcium. Lactate dehydrogenase should be measured; elevated levels

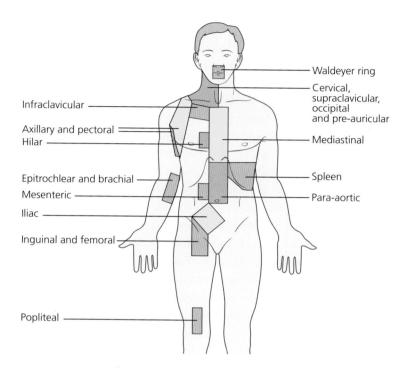

Figure 4.5 The anatomic positions of lymphoid tissue.

have been found to be an adverse prognostic marker at presentation of lymphoma.

Paraproteins are a common finding in B-cell indolent lymphomas and are detected by serum electrophoresis. The proteins are clonal (i.e. they are identical in structure) and are usually immunoglobulin (Ig) G, IgA or IgM, thus reflecting the clonal nature of the tumor and the normal function of the B cells from which the tumor derives. Monitoring paraprotein levels is a useful measure of disease response, especially in certain types of lymphoma such as Waldenström macroglobulinemia/lymphoplasmacytoid lymphoma. Occasionally, the paraprotein may be active against normal cellular components or indeed other proteins in the blood. A paraprotein active against nerve tissue (myelin or axonal) can lead to a peripheral neuropathy or, if it targets red blood cells, may cause hemolytic anemia. Some abnormal proteins may precipitate in colder temperatures, leading to alterations in blood flow, or form immune complexes – cryoglobulins.

Virology. Some centers routinely screen every new patient with lymphoma for HIV, while others restrict screening to patients with known risk factors. However, it is well documented that restricting tests to those with risk factors will miss some HIV-infected individuals. A complete virological screen including hepatitis B and C should be performed.

Staging system. From the results of imaging and bone-marrow biopsy, the lymphoma can be staged by the Ann Arbor system as follows (Figure 4.6):
- stage I: involvement of a single group of lymph nodes
- stage II: involvement of two or more lymph-node groups on the same side of the diaphragm
- stage III: involvement of lymph-node groups on both sides of the diaphragm
- stage IV: widespread disease, often with bone-marrow involvement.

Staging also takes into account the presence of 'B symptoms'.

B symptoms are:
- objectively documented fever
- more than 10% weight loss in 6 months
- night sweats that drench and wake the patient.

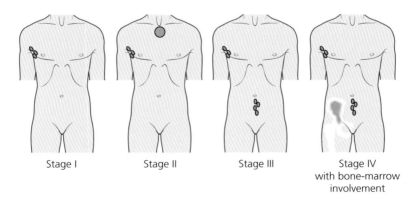

Stage I   Stage II   Stage III   Stage IV
with bone-marrow
involvement

Figure 4.6 Staging of lymphoma.

Absence of B symptoms makes the patient stage A. So, for example, if a patient has drenching night sweats, and has lymphoma in the supraclavicular and mediastinal lymph nodes, but nothing below the diaphragm, the stage is IIB.

Treatment

Once the diagnosis is established and the staging investigations are completed, the patient and relatives need to be fully informed of the nature of the condition and the likely treatment plan. It is important to provide the following:

- verbal and written information about the disorder and its treatment
- information about support organizations
- opportunities to answer questions.
  Treatment options may include:
- chemotherapy (single agent or combination)
- radiotherapy
- immunotherapy using either bioengineered monoclonal antibodies (e.g. rituximab) or cellular immune therapy
- high-dose therapy with stem-cell support.

As lymphomas are spread by the bloodstream and by lymphatic drainage at an early stage, chemotherapy is the mainstay of treatment. Surgery has almost no role except for obtaining tissue for diagnosis or, occasionally, to remove a site of resectable disease that is causing or may cause a life-threatening complication, for example a local bowel tumor that may perforate.

Chemotherapy is thought to kill fractions of the tumor burden at a time. Compounds active against lymphomas are usually combined with other chemotherapy agents to increase efficacy and decrease the chance of resistance. Combination chemotherapy generally improves the response rate compared with single-agent treatment. Several drugs are active against lymphoma but perhaps the best known combination is CHOP. CHOP was first described as an effective therapy for NHL in the late 1970s. This regimen, which is given every 3 weeks, was found to cure about 40% of cases of aggressive lymphoma. Several other drugs were added in later trials, but it was difficult to prove that any of these more elaborate and more toxic regimens conferred any benefit in improving survival rates. CHOP therefore remained the standard of care until the introduction of the monoclonal antibody rituximab in the late 1990s.

Rituximab binds to the CD20 molecule on the surface of B cells, leading to cell death. R-CHOP, as the combination of rituximab and CHOP chemotherapy has become known, saves one additional life for every 10 patients treated compared with CHOP alone and has now become the standard of care for diffuse large B-cell lymphoma.

Indolent lymphomas, such as follicular lymphoma, are not curable with conventional chemotherapy. Treatment is palliative and aims to reduce symptoms and prevent critical organ failure (see Chapter 6, page 69). It is entirely reasonable to monitor the patient (often known as active surveillance) and to intervene only when symptoms appear.

Single-agent oral chemotherapy, such as alkylating agents, can be effective in inducing a partial response and thereby improve the patient's symptoms and general wellbeing. Combination chemotherapy with rituximab will induce a higher response rate and a higher complete remission rate, which appears to translate into increased overall survival.

Ongoing research is also investigating possible new cures for indolent lymphomas, such as reduced intensity conditioning allogeneic stem-cell transplantation (see page 126).

Aggressive lymphomas, such as diffuse large B-cell, lymphoblastic and Burkitt lymphoma, must always be treated with chemotherapy (see pages 55–67). Being rapidly progressive and widely disseminated at the time of initial presentation, local radiotherapy alone has no place, even in the earliest stages of the disease. Burkitt lymphoma is a unique cancer because every cell is undergoing division. Treatment of this disorder requires multi-agent, daily chemotherapy including high-dose methotrexate and cytosine arabinoside, which cross the blood–brain barrier, to protect the central nervous system.

Hodgkin lymphoma was one of the first cancers to be cured by radiotherapy and, in more advanced cases, one of the first cancers to be cured by chemotherapy (see page 109). Like most lymphomas, Hodgkin lymphomas are radiosensitive, so radiotherapy can be useful when the disease is localized (stages IA and IIA), though it is usually given in combination with chemotherapy. Advanced Hodgkin lymphoma (stages IIB–IV) must be treated with combination chemotherapy. The current standard chemotherapy regimen is ABVD.

Modern therapeutic regimens aim to reduce the exposure of patients with early-stage disease to both chemotherapy and radiotherapy by using abbreviated treatment programs and attempting to eliminate radiotherapy altogether.

Management of side effects

Emesis. Many chemotherapy drugs can cause emesis, but the development of highly effective antiemetic drugs, particularly the 5-hydroxytryptamine-3 antagonists, has reduced this complication considerably. Cyclophosphamide, a drug commonly used in the management of lymphoma, causes delayed emesis and antiemetic medication may be needed for 3 or 4 days, rather than the usual 1 or 2 days.

Neuropathy. Peripheral neuropathy is a particular problem with the vinca alkaloid group (vincristine and vinblastine). Other drugs, such as the platinum-based drugs, may also cause neuropathy. The longest nerves are most affected; thus, the tips of the fingers and toes are affected first. Reduction in the dose or discontinuation of the offending vinca alkaloid may be essential.

Mood changes are an important problem with corticosteroid-based chemotherapy. Patients with a history of depressive or other mental illness are particularly at risk. Some patients may become psychotic and require expert psychiatric management.

Hair loss occurs with several chemotherapy drugs. Cyclophosphamide and anthracyclines (doxorubicin, daunorubicin) commonly lead to almost complete alopecia. A cold cap to cool the scalp and restrict blood reaching the follicles is not usually advised during the delivery of chemotherapy for lymphoma because of the way lymphomas are thought to spread; reducing the blood supply to the scalp may protect some disseminating malignant cells from being exposed to the chemotherapy agents administered.

Fertility. The impact of chemotherapy on fertility is important and must be discussed before treatment starts. All men receiving chemotherapy who may wish to have children should be given the option of sperm storage. For women, preserving fertility is more complex and is a function of age, the nature of the underlying disease and properties of the specific chemotherapy regimen. The most commonly used method of preserving fertility in women is cryopreservation of fertilized ova. However, this technique requires 2 weeks of hormonal stimulation and is therefore only possible in those cases in which treatment can be delayed. Furthermore, the technique requires the presence of a willing partner. Other techniques under investigation include oocyte storage, cryopreservation of ovarian tissue and hormone suppression therapy.

Both the type and the dosing regimen of chemotherapy determine the impact of treatment on fertility. Alkylating agents pose the highest risk of infertility, particularly when given daily. Single doses of alkylating drugs, such as melphalan given during high-dose therapy, do not necessarily lead to infertility. CHOP and ABVD rarely cause sterility in either men or women, but women do become more susceptible as they approach the menopause.

Management of bone-marrow suppression. A very important aspect of the delivery of chemotherapy is the likely effect on the patient's normal blood count. Anemia can be corrected by simple red-cell transfusion, although it must be remembered that patients with Hodgkin lymphoma, patients receiving high-dose chemotherapy and those who have received a purine analog (e.g. fludarabine, cladribine) require irradiated blood products in order to prevent the very rare complication of transfusion-associated graft-versus-host disease. Patients with low platelet counts can be given platelet transfusions.

The most serious short-term effect of chemotherapy is to lower the white cell count, most importantly the neutrophil count. Neutrophils have an important function in protecting and maintaining mucosal surfaces such as the lining of the gastrointestinal tract. Loss of neutrophils is accompanied by mucosal ulceration leading to life-threatening Gram-negative bacterial infection. Patients who develop a fever following chemotherapy need urgent assessment and may require admission to hospital to receive intravenous antibiotics.

Response to chemotherapy

The response to chemotherapy determines the subsequent management of the patient. For any curative strategy, a complete response is required.

One way of achieving this in patients with aggressive B-cell lymphomas is to administer four courses of R-CHOP followed by restaging (CT scan and bone-marrow biopsy if indicated; PET scanning is being evaluated for restaging). The outcome will then determine subsequent therapy as follows:

- complete remission (no residual tumor detected on routine staging): patient receives two further courses
- partial remission (at least 50% response to treatment): patient receives two further courses and is restaged
- no response: alternative (salvage/refractory) chemotherapy indicated
- progressive disease: alternative (salvage/refractory) chemotherapy indicated.

With low-grade or indolent lymphomas it is usually only necessary to treat to maximal response. An alternative approach is simply to administer all the courses of chemotherapy and then to assess response at the end of treatment.

Residual masses. One of the central dilemmas of lymphoma management is the interpretation of residual masses following chemotherapy (Figure 4.7).

Not all residual masses that are present after chemotherapy or radiotherapy contain active disease. Indeed, 60% of patients with Hodgkin lymphoma are found to have residual masses on completion of chemotherapy. It is likely that a non-malignant inflammatory infiltrate and fibrotic reaction is responsible. PET scanning may help identify those masses that contain active lymphoma and therefore require more therapy; the technique is, however, still being evaluated and is not 100% reliable. Alternatively, a repeat CT scan a few weeks later will often provide the same information. Clearly, if there is active lymphoma, the mass will usually have grown.

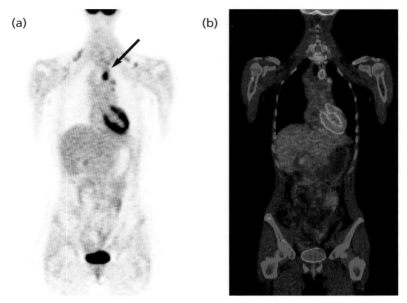

Figure 4.7 (a) PET scan of a patient with a residual mediastinal mass after treatment for Hodgkin lymphoma with recurrence of symptoms. Note the area of greater uptake of radiolabeled glucose in the mediastinum (arrowed). (b) Overlay of CT and PET scan showing that a region of greater uptake is located within a mediastinal mass. Note: heart and brain normally take up more glucose than other organs; the bladder is also highlighted due to excretion of the tracer. (Published with kind permission of Dr F Gleeson, University of Oxford, UK.)

Relapse

The management principles described above should also be followed at relapse. Biopsy is usually recommended to ensure that the lymphoma has not changed. Indolent lymphomas may transform into aggressive lymphomas, and aggressive lymphomas may relapse with previously hidden indolent low-grade disease. Biopsy must be followed by full staging.

Patients who relapse after initial therapy will usually be given a different chemotherapy regimen. For aggressive lymphomas the intention remains curative. In this situation, patients will usually be offered platinum-based chemotherapy (see pages 58 and 60) followed by high-dose therapy and stem-cell rescue. Not surprisingly, relapse therapy is usually associated with a lower response rate.

For indolent lymphomas, relapse may or may not require active therapy. If required, treatment with a different class or combination of chemotherapy is administered. The aim is to relieve symptoms and reduce tumor bulk, and not usually to achieve complete remission. However, a more aggressive approach may be indicated in younger patients.

Key points – general approach to management

- Lymphomas are classified into Hodgkin and non-Hodgkin lymphomas.
- Non-Hodgkin lymphomas are classified into B-cell, T-cell and natural-killer cell types.
- Biopsy and staging are mandatory in the management of lymphoma.
- Lymphomas are often widespread at presentation.
- Chemotherapy is the mainstay of management.
- Neutropenic sepsis is a life-threatening complication of chemotherapy and requires urgent assessment.
- Fertility is an important consideration in any patient of childbearing age receiving chemotherapy or radiotherapy.
- Patients who relapse will be considered for re-biopsy and complete restaging.

Key references

Burton C, Ell P, Linch D. The role of PET imaging in lymphoma. *Br J Haematol* 2004;126:772–84.

Hancock BW, Selby PJ, Maclennan K et al. *Malignant Lymphoma.* Oxford: Oxford University Press, 2001.

Jaffe ES, Harris NL, Stein H, Vardiman JW. *World Health Organization Classification of Tumours. Pathology and Genetics of Tumours of Haematopoietic and Lymphoid Tissues.* Lyon: IARC Press, 2001.

The aggressive B-cell lymphomas (also known as high-grade B-cell lymphomas) include diffuse large B-cell lymphoma (DLBCL), mediastinal large B-cell lymphoma, Burkitt lymphoma and lymphoblastic lymphoma or acute lymphoblastic leukemia (see page 88). Left untreated, these tumors can rapidly be fatal. Treatment aims to provide a cure, and relapse is associated with a poor prognosis.

Diffuse large B-cell lymphoma

The most common aggressive lymphoma is DLBCL, which accounts for approximately 30% of all cases of non-Hodgkin lymphoma (NHL). Typically, the cells are large (Figure 5.1) and express B-cell markers. While there are a few recurring cytogenetic and molecular abnormalities, they are not particularly helpful diagnostically (Table 5.1). Importantly for treatment, most DLBCL express CD20, which is the target for rituximab. The condition may present at any age, but is increasingly common in later life.

Pathology. The most common finding is sheets of large cells which stain with the B-cell markers CD19, CD79a and CD20. Molecular profiling using expression microarrays (see page 37) has identified

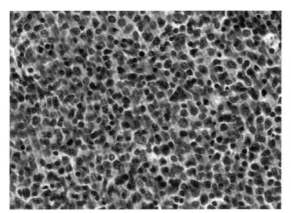

Figure 5.1
Hematoxylin–eosin stained section of diffuse large B-cell lymphoma showing sheets of large, pleomorphic, malignant lymphoid cells.

TABLE 5.1

Characteristics of diffuse large B-cell lymphoma

- Most common high-grade lymphoma
- Usually nodal but also frequently extranodal
- B symptoms common
- Overall, 50% cured with combination chemotherapy
- Pathology reveals sheets of large, pleomorphic B cells
- Immunophenotype CD19+, CD20+, CD79a+, surface IgM+, CD10+/−, *Bcl2*+/−, *Bcl6*+/−

two main types of DLBCL, namely those derived from germinal-center B cells (GCB type) and those derived from a different stage in the B-cell life cycle – so-called non-germinal-center B cells (non-GCB type).

In accordance with their germinal-center derivation, *Bcl6* and CD10 are expressed in about 50% of cases. There is some evidence that the molecular subtype has prognostic significance. The non-GCB subtype has been found to confer a worse prognosis though this observation needs to be verified in a prospective clinical trial.

Clinical presentation. Clinically there are some important considerations.
- About 50% of all cases involve extranodal sites.
- Approximately 30% of patients have underlying indolent B-cell lymphomas.
- DLBCL are aggressive, but approximately 50% are curable with combination chemotherapy.
- 5% will relapse in the central nervous system.

Management of DLBCL, as with all lymphomas, starts with staging. Although outcome is partly dependent on the extent of disease at presentation, treatment is usually with combination chemotherapy, such as R-CHOP, regardless of clinical stage. Staging is, however, crucial, because it is important to identify all the sites involved so that response during therapy can be properly assessed.

Staging investigations include:
- computed tomography (CT) scans of chest, abdomen and pelvis; extranodal sites may need to be reimaged if not adequately visualized
- bone-marrow biopsy
- complete blood count, renal and liver profile, and immunoglobulins
- lactate dehydrogenase (LDH)
- virology, which should include hepatitis B and HIV.

Prognosis can be usefully predicted using the International Prognostic Index (IPI). Patients may be divided into four outcome groups depending on their score (Table 5.2):
- low risk
- low–intermediate risk
- high–intermediate risk
- high risk.

Clinical trials are under way to determine whether more intensive initial chemotherapy will improve the outcome in the poor prognostic groups; however, retrospective data already exist to describe the impact of rituximab on outcome, and a revised IPI has been proposed – the R-IPI. This defines three prognostic groups (Table 5.3). Prospective confirmation of these data is awaited.

Treatment. The standard treatment for DLBCL is R-CHOP given every 21 days. GELA (*Groupe d'Etude des Lymphomes de l'Adulte*) convincingly demonstrated an overall survival advantage by adding

TABLE 5.2

Impact of the International Prognostic Index (IPI) on survival rates in diffuse large B-cell lymphoma

IPI score	Risk category	5-year survival rate
0 or 1	Low	73%
2	Low–intermediate	51%
3	High–intermediate	43%
4 or 5	High	26%

TABLE 5.3

Impact of rituximab on the International Prognostic Index (R-IPI) and survival rates in diffuse large B-cell lymphoma

R-IPI category	4-year survival rate
Very good	94%
Good	80%
Poor	53%

rituximab to CHOP in the elderly (Figure 5.2). Subsequent trials extended this observation to younger patients. German investigators found that giving CHOP every 14 days without rituximab but with growth-factor support achieved a similar outcome; however, this approach has not been compared directly with R-CHOP in a prospective randomized trial. Trials comparing the length of treatment with R-CHOP (21 days versus 14 days) are ongoing. Regimens administered as continuous infusions, such as dose-adjusted EPOCH-R (EPOCH plus rituximab), are also being evaluated as potentially more active treatments.

Early-stage DLBCL is best managed with abbreviated R-CHOP (i.e. a total of four courses). Some centers will use adjunctive radiotherapy. Those patients who have not achieved complete remission by the completion of their fourth course of R-CHOP may be considered to have refractory disease in this setting, and the possibility of using salvage regimens should be discussed.

Follow-up. Patients who are in complete remission can be followed up in an outpatient clinic. Most centers see their patients every few months during the first 2 years when the chance of relapse is highest. Patients can probably be seen less often after 2 years provided they remain free of disease. Many centers now discharge patients after 5 years.

Relapse or progressive disease. The prognosis for patients who relapse after treatment is generally poor, with approximately only 20–30% of patients rescued with salvage/relapse protocols. Most patients destined

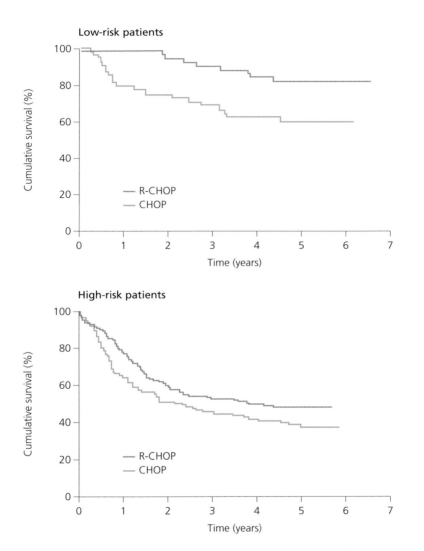

Figure 5.2 Overall survival curves following treatment with CHOP or rituximab plus CHOP in elderly patients. Reprinted with permission from the American Society of Clinical Oncology from Feugier P, Van Hoof A, Sebban C et al. Long-term results of the R-CHOP study in the treatment of elderly patients with diffuse large B-cell lymphoma: a study by the Groupe d'Etude des Lymphomes de l'Adulte. *J Clin Oncol* 2005;23:4117–26.

to relapse will do so in the first 2 years after initial treatment. Salvage protocols vary, but are usually based on regimens containing platinum. The key consideration is response, because patients achieving a satisfactory response may then benefit from high-dose therapy and peripheral stem-cell rescue (Figure 5.3). The following salvage/relapse regimens are used.

- R-DHAP and R-ESHAP are similar regimens given by infusion over 5 days. R-ESHAP is an excellent stem-cell mobilizer, but has a long-term survival rate of only 20% when used as the sole therapeutic agent (i.e. without subsequent high-dose therapy).
- R-ICE is given as an infusion over 3–4 days; like ESHAP, it is a good stem-cell mobilizer.

As suggested above, patients who have relapsed do better if they are able to receive high-dose therapy (see page 123). However, high-dose therapy is only beneficial for patients who achieved a satisfactory response to the initial salvage chemotherapy. Patients who do not respond have chemorefractory disease and are best either entered into clinical trials of novel agents or given palliative care. Occasionally, radiotherapy provides excellent symptomatic relief for localized disease.

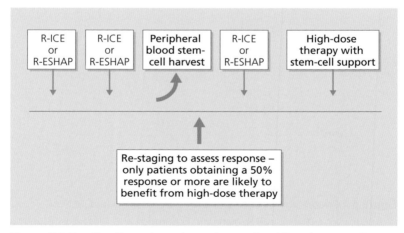

Figure 5.3 Timeline illustrating salvage therapy for diffuse large B-cell lymphoma. Some centers give R-DHAP instead of R-ICE or R-ESHAP. Additional courses are sometimes given to achieve a response before proceeding to high-dose therapy.

Central nervous system prophylaxis. Central nervous system (CNS) involvement is seldom a presenting feature of DLBCL, but does tend to occur at relapse. Patients with involvement of two or more extranodal sites together with a raised LDH are at particular risk of relapse in the CNS. Furthermore, certain anatomic sites may confer risk, such as involvement of the bone marrow, testis, breast, tonsil and paraspinal territory or disease that involves the facial bones and surrounding structures.

This area of lymphoma management is controversial, but most centers invoke some form of prophylaxis for patients thought to be at risk of CNS involvement. Chemotherapy (e.g. methotrexate and cytosine arabinoside) delivered directly into the cerebrospinal fluid by lumbar puncture is one such strategy. An alternative is administration of a sufficiently high dose of systemic drugs to pass the blood–brain barrier (e.g. high-dose methotrexate and high-dose cytosine arabinoside). Addition of intrathecal chemotherapy leads to a greater degree of bone-marrow suppression when combined with standard chemotherapy, and the addition of either high-dose methotrexate or high-dose cytosine arabinoside adds considerably to the toxicity of the regimen.

Burkitt lymphoma

Burkitt lymphoma is a rare, important disease with a distinctive immunophenotype and cytogenetics, which can often be cured with aggressive sequential chemotherapy. Burkitt lymphoma is probably the most aggressive tumor affecting humans. Every cell is undergoing cell division, leading to potentially devastating presentations with huge tumor burdens. There are two main types: endemic Burkitt lymphoma, which is almost always associated with Epstein–Barr virus (EBV) infection; and sporadic Burkitt lymphoma, which occurs more often in Western Europe and the USA, is not as frequently associated with EBV and requires aggressive chemotherapy (Table 5.4).

Pathology. Biopsy of an affected lymph node or other involved tissue will show sheets of small- to medium-sized lymphoid cells with a so-called 'starry-sky' appearance caused by the presence of phagocytic

TABLE 5.4

Characteristics of Burkitt lymphoma

- Endemic or sporadic (which includes HIV-associated)
- Highly aggressive, with 100% proliferation index
- Commonly extranodal: bone marrow, brain, breast, gastrointestinal tract, ovary/testis
- Pathology comprises small, monotonous lymphocytic infiltrate with 'starry-sky' appearance
- Immunophenotype: CD19+, CD20+, CD10+, TdT-, Bcl-2-, sIgM+
- Cytogenetics: t(8;14), t(2;8) or t(8;22)

macrophages dotted about within the tumor (Figure 5.4). These findings are not diagnostic, because they are occasionally seen in other lymphomas. However, the near-100% mitotic rate (as measured by an immunostain such as Ki-67) is not found in any other type of cancer. The immunophenotype is one of a mature germinal-center B-cell phenotype expressing CD19, CD20 and CD10. The extreme mitotic rate is in part due to overexpression of the *c-MYC* oncogene, which forces the cell to proliferate. The gene is located on chromosome 8 and can translocate to one of three immunoglobulin genes located on chromosomes 14, 22 and 2 (t(8;14), t(8;22) or t(2;8)). This places *c-MYC* under the control of the immunoglobulin gene enhancer, thus driving expression.

Clinical presentation. Many patients present with rapidly enlarging lymph nodes, but the disease is almost always widespread and should be treated as such. Extranodal involvement is very common; extensive bone-marrow infiltration, and CNS, ovarian, gastrointestinal and breast involvement are all well recognized. Occasionally, patients will present with florid leukemia. The large tumor bulk often seen in these patients is reflected in very high levels of LDH in some cases. Full staging is mandatory and should include analysis of the cerebrospinal fluid.

Treatment. Burkitt lymphoma requires treatment with high-dose sequential chemotherapy. Effective treatment regimens expose the malignant and rapidly dividing cells to longer periods of chemotherapy than would be achieved with simple CHOP. Another important component of therapy is CNS-directed treatment, usually in the form of high-dose methotrexate or high-dose cytosine arabinoside. Cure rates of 65–80% can be achieved when sequential chemotherapy is delivered

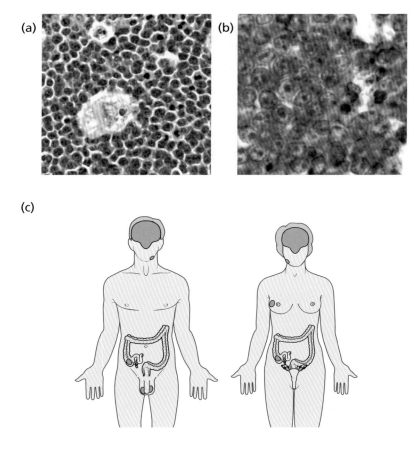

Figure 5.4 Burkitt lymphoma. (a) Hematoxylin–eosin stained section showing a 'starry-sky' appearance. (b) A CD10+ immunostain reflecting the germinal-center origin. (c) Common sites of presentation: brain, jaw, breast, gastrointestinal tract, testis and ovary.

such as CODOX-M or, for higher-risk patients (high LDH and advanced stage), CODOX-M/IVAC. These regimens contain high-dose methotrexate and/or high-dose cytosine arabinoside to protect or treat the CNS. Because of the large bulk at presentation and the rapid response to chemotherapy, steps must be taken to avoid the clinical consequences of killing tumor cells too quickly (tumor lysis syndrome): adequate hydration of the patient with careful recording of fluid balance is essential, along with regular monitoring of renal and cardiac function and electrolytes, and administration of an agent to prevent deposition of uric acid, such as rasburicase (recombinant uric acid oxidase), in the kidneys.

Burkitt-like lymphoma

Burkitt-like lymphoma is probably not a true Burkitt lymphoma, but a variant of DLBCL with a very high proliferation rate. In the World Health Organization (WHO) classification, Burkitt-like lymphoma is defined as having immunophenotypic and cytogenetic criteria for Burkitt lymphoma, but atypical morphology. In practice, the term is often used to describe cases of aggressive B-cell lymphoma with a proliferation fraction close to 100% irrespective of cytogenetic changes. Many clinicians treat Burkitt-like lymphoma with a Burkitt chemotherapy protocol.

Primary mediastinal (thymic) large B-cell lymphoma

Primary mediastinal (thymic) large B-cell lymphoma is a rare, aggressive, locally invasive lymphoma that presents in young adults and more commonly in women. It was once considered a variant of diffuse large-cell lymphoma, but it is now listed as a separate entity in the WHO classification.

Pathology. Mediastinal large B-cell lymphoma is thought to arise from thymic B cells and is characterized by the presence of medium or large lymphoma cells with clear cytoplasm enmeshed in a variable amount of reactive fibrosis (Figure 5.5, Table 5.5). Mediastinal large B-cell lymphoma presents a fairly distinct immunophenotype. The cells express the B-cell antigens CD20, CD19 and CD79a, and may also

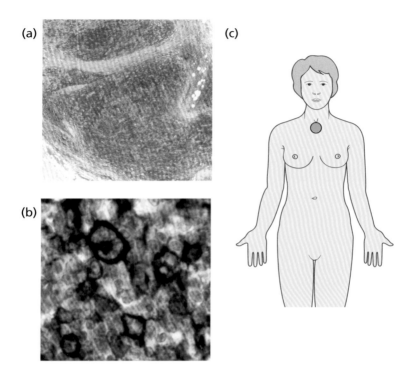

Figure 5.5 Mediastinal large B-cell lymphoma. (a) Low-power hematoxylin–eosin stained section showing prominent fibrosis. (b) A high-power view of CD30 stain. (c) Common site of presentation: mediastinum.

TABLE 5.5

Characteristics of primary mediastinal large B-cell lymphoma

- Typically affects young women
- Locally invasive mediastinal mass
- Symptoms of cough, breathlessness, superior vena caval obstruction
- Pathology comprises large malignant B cells with variable amount of fibrosis
- Immunophenotype: CD19+, CD20+, CD30+, CD10-
- Better prognosis than diffuse large B-cell lymphoma

express CD30, which is better known as a marker of Hodgkin lymphoma. Characteristically, the cells do not express surface immunoglobulin, CD10 or human leukocyte antigen class I molecules. Furthermore, unlike DLBCL, primary B-cell mediastinal lymphomas do not show rearrangements of either the *Bcl2* or *Bcl6* genes. Interestingly, gene-expression microarray studies show that the signature of mediastinal large B-cell lymphoma is more similar to that of classical Hodgkin lymphoma than that of DLBCL.

Cytogenetics of mediastinal large B-cell lymphoma show a characteristic pattern of genomic aberrations with gains on the short arm of chromosomes 9 and 2 (involving the *Jak2* and *c-rel* genes, respectively).

Clinical presentation reflects the fact that this tumor tends to remain localized to the upper anterior mediastinum (Figure 5.6), is aggressive and will invade local structures. Obstruction of the superior vena cava

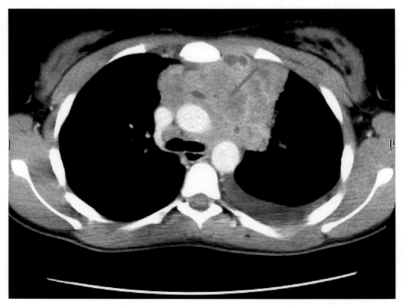

Figure 5.6 Computed tomography scan showing mediastinal large B-cell lymphoma (arrow) in a 20-year-old woman presenting with cervical lymphadenopathy, cough and shortness of breath.

causing cough, dyspnea and stridor is a relatively common clinical presentation. Phrenic nerve palsy or recurrent laryngeal nerve palsy may occur as a direct result of local tissue invasion.

Treatment. Recent studies have found that primary mediastinal large B-cell lymphoma has a favorable outcome compared with DLBCL. Most centers treat mediastinal large B-cell lymphoma using a DLBCL protocol (R-CHOP), though others may use infusional regimens based on the excellent outcome data with dose-adjusted EPOCH-R. Whether the addition of radiotherapy to the mediastinum at the completion of chemotherapy confers survival advantage is controversial. Some centers routinely administer radiotherapy to residual masses, while others reserve radiotherapy for treatment at relapse or progression after salvage and high-dose therapy.

Key points – aggressive B-cell lymphomas

- The commonest aggressive B-cell lymphoma is diffuse large B-cell lymphoma (DLBCL).
- Approximately 50% of DLBCL are curable with R-CHOP.
- Patients who relapse require salvage chemotherapy and, if chemosensitive, will benefit from high-dose chemotherapy and stem-cell rescue.
- Burkitt and Burkitt-like lymphoma have a proliferation rate close to 100% and should be treated with sequential chemotherapy incorporating central nervous system prophylaxis.

Key references

Blum KA, Lozanski G, Byrd JC. Adult Burkitt leukemia and lymphoma. *Blood* 2004;104:3009–20.

Coiffier B, Lepage E, Briere J et al. CHOP chemotherapy plus rituximab compared with CHOP alone in elderly patients with diffuse large-B-cell lymphoma. *N Engl J Med* 2002;346:235–42.

Philip T, Guglielmi C, Hagenbeek A et al. Autologous bone marrow transplantation as compared with salvage chemotherapy in relapses of chemotherapy-sensitive non-Hodgkin's lymphoma. *N Engl J Med* 1995;333:1540–5.

Sweetenham JW. Diffuse large B-cell lymphoma: risk stratification and management of relapsed disease. *Hematology Am Soc Hematol Educ Program* 2005:252–9.

Modern classifications of lymphoma divide non-Hodgkin lymphoma (NHL) into B-cell and T-cell lymphomas. However, the old-fashioned broad division of NHLs into low- and high-grade disease remains clinically useful as it predicts the natural history and clinical behavior of a particular case. Further division into specific entities is based on morphology, immunophenotype, cytogenetics, molecular genetics and clinical behavior. Indolent lymphoma (also known as low-grade lymphoma) is generally considered to be incurable and treatment is used to reduce systemic symptoms or debulk a high tumor burden.

Nearly all low-grade lymphomas are of B-cell origin although occasional T-cell lymphomas, such as angio-immunoblastic lymphoma, can behave in an indolent fashion. The most common low-grade B-cell lymphomas are:

- follicular lymphoma
- mantle cell lymphoma
- marginal zone lymphoma
- lymphoplasmacytoid lymphoma
- small lymphocytic lymphoma
- hairy cell leukemia (which is not discussed in further detail).

Most patients with indolent lymphomas die of their disease. Periods of disease stability are followed by periods of disease progression, which may or may not require treatment depending on symptoms, critical organ involvement or indeed whether the disease bulk is uncomfortable or unsightly. Even when treatment has been particularly effective and the disease is not obvious on a computed tomography scan or bone-marrow biopsy, indicating complete remission, the underlying disorder always remains and disease progression is inevitable.

Follicular lymphoma

Follicular lymphoma is a common, usually nodal, lymphoma with a relatively high rate of transformation to high-grade disease (Table 6.1). It is one of the commonest forms of low-grade B-cell NHL, representing

TABLE 6.1

Characteristics of follicular lymphoma

- Disorder of older people
- Indolent; median survival 8–10 years
- Widespread lymphadenopathy
- Hepatosplenomegaly and bone-marrow involvement common
- Pathology: distorted follicular pattern in lymph node; paratrabecular infiltrate of marrow
- Immunophenotype: CD19+, CD20+, CD10+, Bcl2+
- Cytogenetics: t(14;18)

25% of all lymphoma cases. The disorder affects women as commonly as men and, though it is occasionally seen in young adults, is generally a disorder that affects older people.

Pathology. The malignant cells are small lymphocytes in which aberrant expression of *Bcl2* is driven by the specific translocation t(14;18). They are thought to derive from a germinal-center B cell within lymph-node follicles (see Figure 2.3, page 21). The vastly increased numbers and expanded neoplastic follicles cause complete effacement of the normal lymph-node architecture and create the diagnostic appearance. While the diagnosis of follicular lymphoma is usually straightforward, differentiation from simple reactive so-called follicular hyperplasia may be difficult and requires additional staining using appropriate antibodies. Further diagnostic information can, if needed, be obtained by cytogenetic and molecular analysis.

The diagnostic and characteristic chromosomal translocation, t(14;18), found in this disorder leads to increased amounts of the anti-apoptotic protein Bcl2 within the abnormal lymphocytes (not found in reactive germinal centers). This confers a survival advantage on the neoplastic cells. Thus, the finding of Bcl2+ abnormal lymphocytes within expanded lymph-node follicles is strong evidence for the specific diagnostic translocation and therefore the diagnosis of follicular lymphoma.

Follicular lymphoma in the bone marrow presents as a characteristic paratrabecular infiltrate. As expected, the neoplastic infiltrate is Bcl2+. Occasionally, in more aggressive cases, the neoplastic lymphocytes appear in the peripheral blood, where they appear as darkly stained abnormal cleaved lymphoid cells.

As part of the pathological assessment, the number of large, immature-looking cells (called centroblasts) are counted and the follicular lymphoma divided into three grades:
- grade I (< 5 centroblasts per high-power field)
- grade II (5–10 centroblasts per high-power field)
- grade III (> 10 centroblasts per high-power field).

Grade III is often thought to be more aggressive and may be treated as a diffuse large B-cell lymphoma (see page 55). However, this grading system is necessarily subjective, and its clinical significance is therefore uncertain.

The immunophenotype of the B-cell derived from a neoplastic germinal center in follicular lymphoma expresses the ubiquitous B-cell markers CD19 and CD20, but the germinal-center marker CD10 and positive staining for Bcl2 are more specific (Figure 6.1).

Transformation into diffuse high-grade NHL is not uncommon and may occur in up to 60% of cases, conferring a poor prognosis.

Clinical presentation. Although many patients present with painless enlargement of lymph nodes, most are found to have widespread disease after staging. Bone-marrow involvement is found in 60–80% of cases, and splenomegaly is also common. Extranodal disease is rare, but does occur and can affect various organs, including the skin and the gastrointestinal tract.

The disease course is one of periods of stability followed by periods of progression that may require treatment; the intervals between interventions become progressively shorter (Figure 6.2).

One of the many difficulties in managing follicular lymphoma is its uncertain prognosis: some patients survive for more than 10 years, while others die within 2 or 3 years of presentation. The uncertainty surrounding the prognosis of follicular lymphoma has been clarified by the recent development of the Follicular Lymphoma International

71

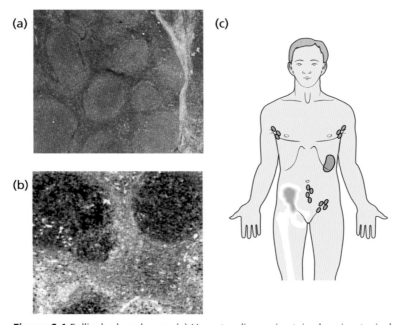

Figure 6.1 Follicular lymphoma. (a) Hematoxylin–eosin stain showing typical distorted follicular structure of an affected lymph node. (b) CD10 stain showing positivity in the germinal center along with scattered interfollicular cells. (c) Common sites of involvement: lymph nodes, spleen (later stages of disease) and bone marrow (common).

Prognostic Index (FLIPI), which has been successfully validated (Figure 6.3). This clinical scoring system helps to determine which patients are at higher risk and may therefore be eligible for experimental or aggressive therapy. The FLIPI adds one point for each of the following five parameters:

- age 60 years or over
- hemoglobin less than 12 g/dL
- serum lactate dehydrogenase level above the upper limit of normal
- stage III–IV (see page 47)
- more than four nodal sites involved.

Patients who score more than two points would be considered intermediate or high risk. The most feared complication, because it confers such a poor prognosis, is the onset of high-grade transformation.

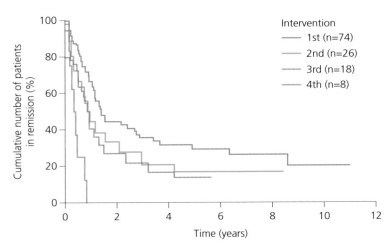

Figure 6.2 The natural history of follicular lymphoma is characterized by progressively shorter remissions in advanced disease. Reprinted with permission from the American Society of Clinical Oncology from Gallagher CJ, Gregory WM, Jones AE et al. Follicular lymphoma: prognostic factors for response and survival. *J Clin Oncol* 1986;4:1470–80.

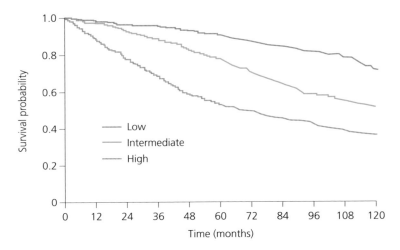

Figure 6.3 The Follicular Lymphoma International Prognostic Index. This research was originally published in *Blood*. Solal-Céligny P et al. Follicular lymphoma international prognostic index. *Blood* 2004;104:1258–65. © American Society of Hematology.

This is usually heralded either by rapidly enlarging nodal disease or by the onset of systemic symptoms, but unfortunately there is no easy way of predicting this yet.

Treatment. Follicular lymphoma is an indolent, slowly progressive disease. Patients should simply be monitored unless there are specific indications for treatment, such as systemic symptoms, critical organ failure or bulky disease. There is no firm evidence that early treatment improves outcome, and the so-called 'watch and wait' approach is entirely reasonable. If treatment is indicated it should ideally be non-toxic. Single-agent chlorambucil or CVP are well-tolerated treatments and used in many countries. The addition of the anti-CD20 monoclonal antibody rituximab improves response rates and has been found to double the time to disease progression from 15 to 30 months in a recent trial comparing CVP with R-CVP (Figure 6.4). Furthermore,

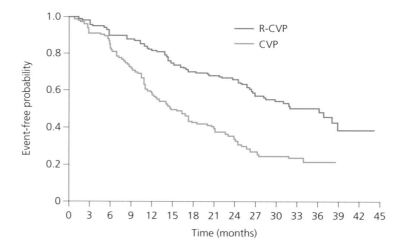

Figure 6.4 Time to progression in patients with follicular lymphoma treated with CVP (median 15 months) versus R-CVP (median 32 months). This research was originally published in *Blood*. Marcus R et al. CVP chemotherapy plus rituximab compared with CVP as first-line treatment for advanced follicular lymphoma. *Blood* 2005;105:1417–23. © American Society of Hematology.

the addition of rituximab to a number of combination chemotherapy regimens has not only been shown to improve response rates and progression-free survival but overall survival as well. Thus, the standard first-line therapy for follicular lymphoma is rituximab with combination chemotherapy, such as R-CVP, R-CHOP or R-FMD. The question remains as to whether more intensive antibody-chemotherapy regimens such as R-CHOP improve survival rates over less intensive regimens such as R-CVP.

For patients with early-stage follicular lymphoma (stage IA or IIA), radiotherapy is also an option. Most low-grade lymphomas are remarkably radiosensitive so that for patients with localized bulky disease this may be the treatment of choice. In fact, some studies suggest that radiotherapy alone may be curative in about 50% of patients with early-stage disease. However, radiotherapy is thought to reduce the chance of successful future stem-cell harvesting, so it is best avoided in younger patients who may need high-dose therapy later.

Patients who progress after first-line therapy can be treated again with the same regimen provided that the duration of their initial response was favorable. Patients whose disease is refractory to first-line therapy will require a second-line treatment, such as CHOP or a fludarabine-containing regimen; the addition of rituximab may also be beneficial.

The addition of maintenance rituximab for patients who have a good partial or complete response to treatment is currently the subject of several randomized clinical trials. One recent trial has shown benefit for relapsed patients treated with CHOP with or without rituximab who went on to receive maintenance rituximab for 2 years at 3-monthly intervals (Figure 6.5).

It is important to note that the treatment-free interval becomes progressively shorter with each relapse (see Figure 6.2, page 73). Therefore, those patients who have been exposed to two or more chemotherapy regimens, and those with rapidly progressing disease, should be considered for experimental procedures such as high-dose therapy with stem-cell rescue, or allografting with reduced-intensity conditioning (see pages 123–6). There is emerging evidence that high-dose therapy with stem-cell rescue may result in prolonged remissions and many centers use this

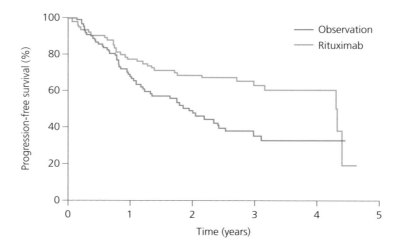

Figure 6.5 Rituximab maintenance treatment is associated with significantly improved progression-free survival in patients who responded initially to CHOP with or without rituximab. This research was originally published in *Blood*. Van Oers MHJ et al. Rituximab maintenance improves clinical outcome of relapsed/resistant follicular non-Hodgkin lymphoma in patients both with and without rituximab during induction: results of a prospective randomized phase 3 intergroup trial. *Blood* 2006;108: 3295–301. © American Society of Hematology.

approach for patients who undergo high-grade transformation or whose remissions are short with standard regimens.

Mantle cell lymphoma

Mantle cell lymphoma is an aggressive low-grade NHL representing 4–8% of all lymphomas; it has the worst outcome of any of the B-cell lymphomas. It presents in middle age or later life, predominantly affects men and has a propensity to involve the gastrointestinal tract (Table 6.2).

Pathology. Mantle cell lymphoma arises from small, atypical lymphoid cells in the mantle zone of secondary lymphoid follicles. Thus, though the appearance of affected lymph nodes is very variable, the greatly

TABLE 6.2

Characteristics of mantle cell lymphoma

- Middle-aged and older men
- Short median survival of 3–4 years
- Widespread lymphadenopathy; splenomegaly, and bone-marrow and gastrointestinal involvement common
- Pathology: distorted follicular or diffuse pattern made up of small lymphocytes
- Immunophenotype: CD19+, CD20+, CD5+, cyclin D1+
- Cytogenetics: t(11;14)

expanded abnormal mantle zones surrounding the lymph-node follicles are characteristic. The cells express the usual B-cell markers, CD19 and CD20, but are characteristically CD5+, a feature shared only with B-cell chronic lymphocytic leukemia (CLL). The diagnosis is confirmed by the finding of cyclin D1+ cells in paraffin sections. The molecule cyclin D1, which is responsible for driving the cells into the cell cycle, is the product of the underlying translocation t(11;14), which is specific for mantle cell lymphoma and which can be identified using standard cytogenetic techniques and fluorescent in-situ hybridization (Figure 6.6).

Clinical presentation. The characteristic presenting complaint is progressive painless lymphadenopathy with surprisingly few systemic symptoms. Staging investigations usually reveal widespread disease involving the spleen, bone marrow and, not uncommonly, abnormal circulating cells in the blood. Extranodal disease in the form of gastrointestinal involvement (lymphomatous polyposis) is common and has been reported in up to 80% of cases in some series. Most series report response rates of 60–80% but remission duration of only 2–3 years, and the median survival is 3–4 years. Some cases, however, can be surprisingly indolent. Low Ki67 expression may be associated with this group of patients.

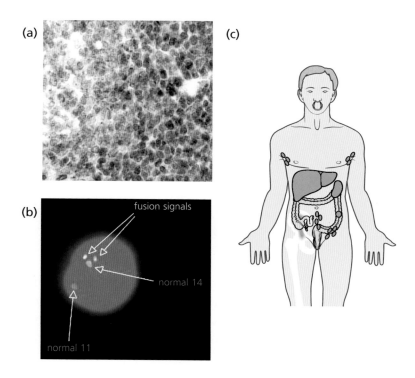

Figure 6.6 Mantle cell lymphoma. (a) Cyclin D1 immunostain with positive cells in the mantle zone of the germinal center. (b) Fluorescent in-situ hybridization showing t(11;14). (c) Common sites of presentation: Waldeyer ring, spleen (60%), large segments of bowel (60%), lymph nodes (generalized; 90%), bone marrow (almost always) and blood (30%).

Treatment. Most patients are treated with combination chemotherapy such as CHOP or combinations of fludarabine and cyclophosphamide. Recently, more intensive multiple drug combinations such as hyperCVAD-MA have been shown to induce longer remissions, which in some series have been consolidated with high-dose therapy and stem-cell rescue or allografting with reduced intensity conditioning (see pages 123–6). The impact of these more intensive approaches is unknown and is the subject of ongoing randomized clinical trials.

Marginal zone lymphoma

Marginal zone lymphomas (Table 6.3) can be divided into three main subtypes:

- extranodal marginal zone lymphoma or lymphoma of mucosa-associated lymphoid tissue (MALT), which typically involves sites such as the stomach, lung, salivary gland and thyroid
- splenic marginal zone lymphoma (equivalent to splenic lymphoma with villous lymphocytosis, SLVL)
- nodal marginal zone lymphoma, which is extremely rare and may simply represent spread of extranodal and splenic marginal zone lymphomas.

Marginal zone lymphomas are strongly associated with both autoimmune disorders (e.g. Hashimoto's thyroiditis and Sjögren's syndrome) and bacterial infection; both represent some form of chronic antigenic stimulation. The link between infectious agents and the development of MALT lymphomas is becoming compelling. *Helicobacter pylori* is the causative agent in most gastric MALT lymphomas and other bacterial agents, such as *Campylobacter jejuni*, may have a role in the pathogenesis of the small-bowel MALT lymphoma formerly known as α-chain disease. Futhermore, the spirochete *Borrelia burgdorferi* has been implicated in cutaneous MALT lymphomas.

TABLE 6.3

Characteristics of marginal zone lymphoma

- Three types of marginal zone lymphoma
  - Nodal (rare)
  - Extranodal (mucosa-associated lymphoid tissue; MALT)
  - Splenic
- Extranodal type often localized and may be cutaneous
- Associated with autoimmune disorders and infection
- Pathology: lymphoepithelioid lesions
- Immunophenotype: CD19+, CD20+, CD5-, CD10-, IgM+, CD23-
- Cytogenetics: t(11;18) in a proportion of gastric MALT

Pathology. The pathology of MALT is difficult. The lymphoma arises in abnormally located islands of lymphoid tissue within glandular structures. It invades tissues such as the stomach mucosa and the thyroid epithelium. The presence of so-called lymphoepitheloid lesions within the tumor is a characteristic feature (Figure 6.7). The abnormal B cells show a tendency towards plasma cell or 'monocytoid' differentiation; in other words, the cells have ample cytoplasm and the nuclear:cytoplasmic ratio is low. While the cells express CD19 and CD20, together with surface immunoglobulin, there is no absolute diagnostic immunophenotype. Splenic marginal zone lymphoma, which

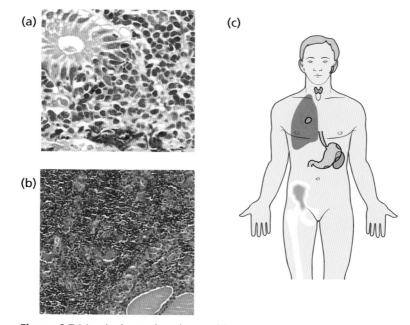

Figure 6.7 Marginal zone lymphoma. (a) Hematoxylin-eosin stain showing a typical lymphoepithelioid lesion in the mucosa-associated lymphoid tissue (MALT) lymphoma subtype. (b) Hematoxylin-eosin stain of MALT lymphoma affecting the thyroid gland with residual thyroid tissue in the bottom right-hand corner. (c) Common sites of presentation: the MALT subtype commonly involves the stomach, lung, thyroid and salivary glands; the splenic subtype commonly involves the spleen and bone marrow.

arises from the marginal zone in the white pulp of the spleen, is often associated with a peripheral blood villous lymphocytosis (SLVL) and a small paraprotein.

Recent research has identified three main cytogenetic abnormalities associated with MALT lymphoma:

- t(11;18)/*API2-MALT1* fusion, which is present in 20–50% of gastric MALT lymphomas and is associated with persistence or recurrence of disease after treatment of *H. pylori* infection
- t(14;18)/*IgH-MALT1* fusion (NB different from follicular lymphoma translocation)
- t(1;14)/*Bcl10-IgH* fusion.

Interestingly in normal cells, both MALT1 and Bcl-10 proteins are involved in the same intracellular signaling pathway linking the antigen receptor (immunoglobulin in B cells, T-cell receptor in T cells) to an important molecule called nuclear factor-κ B. Deregulation of this pathway may well be a common event in the pathogenesis of MALT lymphoma.

Clinical presentation. MALT lymphoma of the stomach is the most common form of marginal zone lymphoma. It mainly affects patients over 50 years of age. The most common presenting complaint is dyspepsia, which may be longstanding and which is often misdiagnosed as simple peptic ulceration or esophagitis. Most cases are associated with *H. pylori* infection which, when eradicated with antibiotic treatment, may lead to spontaneous resolution of symptoms and regression of the tumor. A proportion of gastric MALT lymphomas acquire a novel genetic translocation, t(11;18). These patients tend to have widespread disease, fail to respond to *H. pylori* eradication and have a worse prognosis. High-grade transformation may occur.

Marginal zone lymphomas in other organs such as the salivary glands or the thyroid tend to remain localized and present with simple glandular swelling or local pain. Thyroid marginal zone lymphoma may lead to tracheal compression and stridor.

Cutaneous marginal zone lymphoma, while less frequently seen, still represents one of the commonest forms of skin lymphoma.

Treatment. Marginal zone lymphomas are often localized and local treatments may be curative; for example, radiotherapy to an affected salivary gland or surgical excision of an isolated cutaneous lesion. For tumors known to be associated with antigen stimulation, such as *H. pylori*-driven gastric MALT, eradication of the infectious agent is the first-line treatment, but if this fails chlorambucil may be effective. Trials are under way to determine whether the use of rituximab, either alone or in combination with chemotherapy, provides additional clinical benefits.

Patients with more aggressive disease or those that undergo high-grade transformation require combination chemotherapy such as CHOP. Splenectomy is the treatment of choice for patients with SLVL.

Lymphoplasmacytoid lymphoma/Waldenström macroglobulinemia

Lymphoplasmacytoid lymphoma (LPL) is reported to be a relatively rare, poorly defined, low-grade lymphoma (Table 6.4). However, the condition appears to overlap with other indolent lymphomas, particularly chronic lymphocytic leukemia and the marginal zone lymphomas. LPL affects the middle-aged and elderly. An immunoglobulin (Ig) M paraprotein is characteristic.

TABLE 6.4

Characteristics of lymphoplasmacytoid lymphoma/ Waldenström macroglobulinemia

- Indolent lymphoma
- Incidence increases with age
- Bone-marrow involvement common with associated IgM paraprotein
- Widespread lymphadenopathy and splenomegaly may be present
- Pathology: lymphocytic infiltrate with plasmacytoid features, often with increased numbers of mast cells
- Immunophenotype: CD19+, CD20+, CD5-, CD23-, IgM+, CD10-

Pathology. The diagnosis is usually made from either lymph-node or bone-marrow biopsy. The abnormal neoplastic lymphoid cells have a marked propensity for plasma cell differentiation and an excess of mast cells is often present, which is a helpful diagnostic feature (Figure 6.8). There are almost no specific diagnostic markers for this disease. The cells express CD19 and CD20, but lack CD5 and CD23, which distinguishes them from B-cell CLL, and CD10, which usually excludes follicular lymphoma. An IgM paraprotein, or more rarely another class of paraprotein, is usually found in cases of LPL. There are no specific chromosomal translocations associated with the condition; 6q deletions are perhaps the most commonly reported abnormality. Distinguishing these lymphomas from marginal zone lymphomas is difficult and some authors would consider LPL a variant of marginal cell lymphoma.

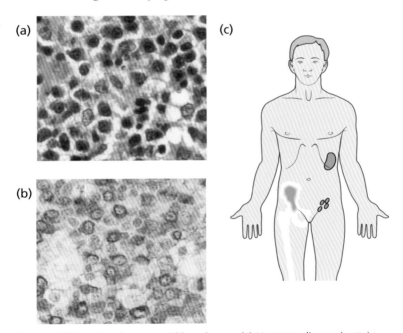

Figure 6.8 Lymphoplasmacytoid lymphoma. (a) Hematoxylin–eosin stain showing typical plasmacytoid appearance of the malignant lymphocytes. (b) An immunostain for λ light chains. (c) Common sites of presentation: spleen, lymph nodes, bone marrow (70–80%) and blood (IgM paraprotein).

Clinical presentation. The most distinctive feature of LPL is the presence of IgM paraprotein, which may determine the clinical presentation as it can lead to hyperviscosity, presenting with headache, visual disturbance and, more dramatically, stroke. The paraprotein may also interfere with clotting mechanisms causing bleeding (e.g. acquired von Willebrand disease), and may even cause various 'autoimmune' phenomena, such as a disabling sensory-motor neuropathy. The paraprotein's physicochemical properties may cause it to precipitate at low temperatures (cryoglobulins), causing acrocyanosis. In all other respects, the presentation is similar to other indolent lymphomas with lymphadenopathy, frequent enlargement of the spleen and liver, and bone-marrow involvement.

Treatment is aimed at alleviating symptoms and is, as with other low-grade lymphoproliferative disorders, seldom curative. Single-agent chlorambucil or fludarabine, or CVP is reasonable first-line therapy. Relapsed disease may require combination chemotherapy, such as CHOP. Rituximab has a response rate of approximately 30% as a single agent, which will increase when combined with chemotherapy. After initial treatment with rituximab, a temporary worsening of paraprotein-mediated phenomena (e.g. peripheral neuropathy) has been reported, which is is thought to be due to the release of antibody following cell lysis. This process has been termed the IgM surge. Patients presenting with hyperviscosity may require urgent plasma exchange to lower the IgM level. Overall survival is thought to be 5–7 years, which is lower than that of follicular lymphoma or CLL.

Small lymphocytic lymphoma/chronic lymphocytic leukemia

Small lymphocytic lymphoma (SLL)/CLL is the most common low-grade B-cell lymphoma (Table 6.5). It often presents incidentally when a lymphocytosis is found on a routine blood count. When the disorder principally affects the peripheral blood, the term chronic lymphocytic (or lymphatic) leukemia is used. The disorder is usually referred to as small lymphocytic lymphoma when there is almost no blood spill and the patient presents with lymphadenopathy.

Pathology. The malignant B cells are usually small, not much bigger than a red cell, and express CD5, CD19 and CD23. Expression of CD38 and ZAP70 confer a poor prognosis, while deletion of 17p defines a group of patients who are chemorefractory. Certain other cytogenetic abnormalities confer a survival advantage, such as deletion of 13q.

Clinical presentation. B-cell CLL characteristically begins with a peripheral blood lymphocytosis. Patients subsequently develop lymphadenopathy followed by hepatosplenomegaly before finally succumbing to bone-marrow failure. At any stage of the disease, autoimmune phenomena such as autoimmune hemolytic anemia and/or immune thrombocytopenic purpura can develop, which may dominate the clinical picture.

Treatment. No treatment is necessary in the early stages of the disease. Later, particularly when there are significant systemic symptoms or signs of bone-marrow failure, chlorambucil or fludarabine will control the disorder. Relapsed disease becomes increasingly difficult to treat, though combinations of fludarabine and cyclophosphamide may

TABLE 6.5

Characteristics of small lymphocytic lymphoma/chronic lymphocytic leukemia

- May be very indolent
- Incidence increases with age; rare under 50 years
- Blood involvement common
- Clinical course starts with lymphocytosis then progresses to lymphadenopathy followed by splenomegaly and finally bone-marrow failure
- Pathology: infiltration by small mature lymphocytes
- Immunophenotype: CD19+, CD5+, CD20 weak, sIg weak, CD23+
- Cytogenetics variable: good prognosis del(13q); poor prognosis del(17p)

Key points – indolent B-cell lymphomas

- Low-grade B-cell lymphomas are more common in the elderly and treatment is usually aimed at alleviating symptoms rather than curing the disease.
- Some low-grade lymphomas, such as follicular and mantle cell lymphoma, have characteristic immunophenotypes and cytogenetics that permit diagnosis.
- Other low-grade lymphomas are hard to diagnose definitively because of the lack of specific markers (e.g. marginal zone and lymphoplasmacytoid lymphoma).
- Knowledge of the cause of the lymphoma has in some cases led to improved treatments (e.g. *Helicobacter pylori* infection and gastric mucosa-associated lymphoid tissue lymphoma).

---

still induce remissions, which potentially offer the option of more experimental curative therapy, such as reduced-intensity conditioning allografting (see page 126).

The anti-CD52 antibody alemtuzumab (also known as CAMPATH-1H) has activity in chemorefractory patients, though bulky disease often does not respond well. Surprisingly, although CD20 expression is classically weak on SLL/CLL cells, rituximab has been used in some regimens and has been shown to improve response rates. However, a routine role for this agent has yet to be defined.

CLL does not run a slow indolent course in all patients. The prognosis is variable and some patients respond poorly to chemotherapy.

Much research has been carried out to define markers of poor prognosis and thereby identify disease that may benefit from more aggressive treatment. An important milestone was the discovery that some patients have somatic hypermutation of the immunoglobulin heavy chain genes, whereas others do not. It is now clear that the unmutated cases are associated with shorter survival. Mutational status is not easy to assess routinely and other factors may act as a surrogate marker, such as the molecule ZAP70. However, perhaps the most important prognostic marker is the presence of del17p (p53 deletion), which predicts a very poor response to chemotherapy, and is an indication for treatment with corticosteroids and the anti-CD52 antibody CAMPATH-1H.

Key references

Hiddemann W, Buske C, Drayling M et al. Current management of follicular lymphomas. *Br J Haematol* 2007;136:191–202.

Khouri IF, Romaguera J, Kantarjian H et al. Hyper-CVAD and high-dose methotrexate/cytarabine followed by stem-cell transplantation: an active regimen for aggressive mantle-cell lymphoma. *J Clin Oncol* 1998;16:3803–9.

Marcus R, Imrie K, Belch A et al. CVP chemotherapy plus rituximab compared with CVP as first-line treatment for advanced follicular lymphoma. *Blood* 2005;105:1417–23.

Montserrat E. New prognostic markers in CLL. *Hematology Am Soc Hematol Educ Program* 2006:279–84.

Thieblemont C. Clinical presentation and management of marginal zone lymphomas. *Hematology Am Soc Hematol Educ Program* 2005:307–13.

Van Oers MH, Klasa R, Marcus RE et al. Rituximab maintenance improves clinical outcome of relapsed/resistant follicular non-Hodgkin lymphoma in patients both with and without rituximab during induction: results of a prospective randomized phase 3 intergroup trial. *Blood* 2006;108:3295–301.

In Europe and the USA, T-cell lymphomas represent about 5% of cases of non-Hodgkin lymphoma. Most T-cell lymphomas are aggressive except for the primary cutaneous forms, such as mycosis fungoides, which can have a protracted and indolent course if they remain localized to the skin. As with B-cell lymphomas, T-cell lymphomas are divided into different clinicopathological entities in terms of cell lineage, immunophenotype, cytogenetics and molecular profile. Tumors derived from natural-killer (NK) cells are very rare and tend to present in the nose and adjacent structures, though occasionally they can present as a frank leukemia.

T cells acquire several identifiable markers during maturation. CD1, CD2 and CD7 are early markers with later expression of CD3, which is associated with the T-cell receptor. CD4 and CD8 are late markers (post-thymic maturation) and define more mature immunocompetent T cells (see Chapter 2).

Precursor T-cell lymphoblastic leukemia/lymphoma

Precursor T-cell lymphoblastic leukemia/lymphoma is an aggressive tumor better known as acute lymphoblastic leukemia (ALL) or lymphoblastic lymphoma (LBL). The tumor is usually defined as LBL when there is no obvious blood involvement and only minimal bone-marrow involvement. The clinical behavior of this disease is very similar to precursor B-cell lymphoblastic leukemia/lymphoma and it typically presents as a large mediastinal mass. T-cell ALL/LBL is more common in adolescents and early adult life, and is rarer in the elderly (Table 7.1).

Pathology. Involved tissues typically contain sheets of blast cells that stain with precursor T-cell markers such as CD34, CD2, CD7, CD3 and TdT (Figure 7.1). Many cases of T-cell ALL/LBL will also stain for CD10. Importantly, these staining characteristics are also evident in cells from readily accessible sites, such as peripheral blood and pleural

TABLE 7.1

Characteristics of T-cell lymphoblastic lymphoma

- Commonly presents in young people
- Mediastinal mass common, but bone-marrow and peripheral-blood involvement also often found
- Pathology: sheets of large, immature lymphoid blast cells
- Immunophenotype: CD10+, TdT+, together with T- or B-cell markers depending on lineage of origin

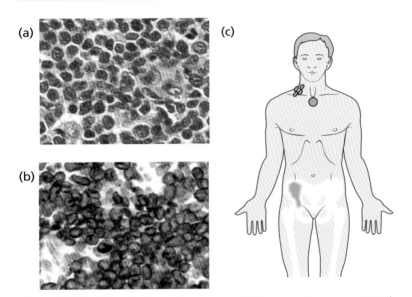

Figure 7.1 T-cell lymphoblastic lymphoma. (a) Hematoxylin–eosin stained section. (b) CD3 immunostain. (c) Common sites of presentation: mediastinum, lymph nodes, blood and bone marrow (common).

effusions, making a formal biopsy under these circumstances unnecessary.

Clinical presentation. Patients with a mediastinal mass commonly present with superior vena caval obstruction, cough or stridor, with or without systemic symptoms. In patients with ALL, fatigue, breathlessness, infection and bleeding are more usual.

89

Treatment. Both LBL and ALL are treated with leukemia protocols. Therapy is administered in three main phases: induction treatment to achieve remission; consolidation therapy including central nervous system (CNS) prophylaxis; and maintenance treatment given over a 2-year period. There is some evidence to support the use of high-dose therapy with stem-cell rescue in patients with LBL following consolidation, rather than proceeding to maintenance treatment. In very young children, cure can often be achieved with combination chemotherapy but, in young adults, the cure rate is lower at about 50%. In older adults, the disorder is associated with a very poor prognosis.

Large granular lymphocyte leukemia

Large granular lymphocyte (LGL) leukemia is one of the few T-cell disorders that typically behaves in an indolent fashion. The disorder is characterized by the presence of increased numbers of large granular lymphocytes in the peripheral blood, autoimmune features (often rheumatoid arthritis) and neutropenia.

Pathology. Unlike the majority of T-cell disorders, LGL is characterized by an expansion of CD8+ lymphocytes, which show obvious pink cytoplasmic granules. Most LGLs also express CD3, but a small proportion express NK markers only (Figure 7.2). The diagnosis is usually made by inspection of peripheral blood in which the presence of LGLs in the context of neutropenia is highly suggestive. Bone-marrow biopsy is less reliable, but may show a similar excess of CD8+ T cells, though their characteristic morphology is less discernible.

Clinical presentation. The clinical manifestations of LGL leukemia are diverse. Some patients present with autoimmune features reminiscent of rheumatoid arthritis, while others will present with neutropenia. There is an overlap between Felty's syndrome (neutropenia and splenomegaly in a patient with rheumatoid arthritis) and LGL leukemia.

Treatment. Patients in whom LGL leukemia is an incidental finding may require no specific therapy. For patients at risk of neutropenic

(a)

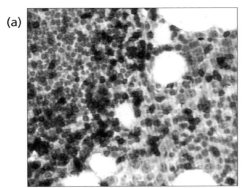

(b)

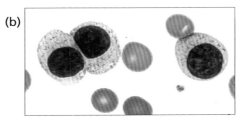

Figure 7.2 Large granular lymphocyte leukemia. (a) CD3 immunostain of bone marrow showing scattered positive cells. (b) Large granular lymphocytes in the peripheral blood.

sepsis, low-dose oral methotrexate or other simple immunosuppressant therapy will improve the neutrophil count. Splenectomy and granulocyte colony-stimulating factor have been reported to be effective in restoring the neutrophil count in some cases.

Adult T-cell leukemia/lymphoma

Adult T-cell lymphoma/leukemia (ATLL) is an aggressive lymphoma associated with human T-cell lymphotropic virus 1 (HTLV-1) infection seen in patients of Afro-Caribbean, Japanese or Southeast Asian origin, where this virus is endemic. HTLV-1 is a retrovirus spread through infected cells in blood, semen and breast milk (Table 7.2).

Pathology. While it is unclear how HTLV-1 causes this lymphoma, the virus infects CD4+ lymphocytes, which leads to upregulation of the interleukin-2 (IL-2) receptor, among many other molecules (Figure 7.3). The characteristic cells of ATLL are medium-sized lymphocytes of which some have polylobated nuclei, sometimes called flower cells. The cells express CD4 and CD25 (IL-2 receptor).

TABLE 7.2

Characteristics of adult T-cell leukemia/lymphoma

- Associated with human T-cell lymphotropic virus 1
- Particularly common in Japan and Caribbean basin
- Commonly presents with lymphadenopathy, hepatosplenomegaly, rash, blood and marrow involvement (flower cells in the smear), hypercalcemia and bone lesions
- Pathology: diffuse infiltration by polymorphic lymphoid cells
- Immunophenotype: CD3+, CD4+, CD5+, CD7-, CD25+

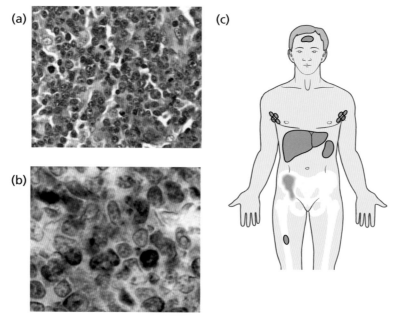

(a) (b) (c)

Figure 7.3 Adult T-cell leukemia/lymphoma. (a) Hematoxylin–eosin stain showing diffuse infiltration by pleomorphic cells. (b) CD4 immunostain. (c) Common sites of presentation: CNS relapse common, liver, spleen, lymph nodes, skin rash, blood, bone marrow and bone.

Clinical presentation. Patients are usually middle-aged and present with widespread lymphadenopathy, enlargement of the liver and spleen, and often skin involvement. In most cases, there is involvement of the peripheral blood and bone marrow, and occasionally the white cell count may be extremely high. Another unusual feature of this disease is the very high prevalence of associated hypercalcemia and, less commonly, lytic bone lesions. CNS involvement is a devastating complication that most often occurs on relapse. The prognosis of ATLL is generally poor and very few patients survive for more than 1–2 years. A small number of patients have disease with a more indolent course.

Treatment. The mainstay of treatment is CHOP chemotherapy and, despite no definite evidence of its efficacy, most patients also receive antiretroviral therapy. The relatively high incidence of CNS involvement at relapse may be an indication for some form of CNS prophylaxis.

Peripheral T-cell lymphoma, unspecified

Peripheral T-cell lymphoma, unspecified, is a rare, clinically aggressive lymphoma with a poor prognosis (Table 7.3). It may be considered as the T-cell equivalent of DLBCL, in that it represents a 'diagnostic dustbin' of otherwise unclassifiable T-cell lymphomas.

Pathology. Most cases exhibit a CD4+ positive T-cell phenotype, though, as with all T-cell lymphomas, there may be much heterogeneity in antigen expression (Figure 7.4).

TABLE 7.3

Characteristics of peripheral T-cell lymphoma, unspecified

- Incidence increases with age
- Aggressive tumor, which often progress on, or shortly after, therapy
- Widespread, small-volume lymphadenopathy and pronounced B symptoms
- Pathology: infiltration with polymorphic malignant T cells
- Immunophenotype: highly variable; CD3+, usually CD4+

Clinical presentation. Most patients are middle-aged or elderly and typically present with widespread, often relatively small-volume, lymphadenopathy with marked systemic symptoms, particularly fever and weight loss.

Treatment is with CHOP or equivalent chemotherapy. In many patients, however, disease progression occurs during treatment, and salvage chemotherapy proceeding to high-dose therapy is required. Some centers treat peripheral T-cell lymphomas with high-dose therapy as part of first-line treatment in view of the poor prognosis.

(a)   (b)

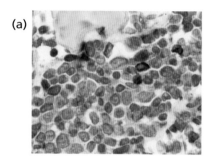

Figure 7.4 Peripheral T-cell lymphoma. (a) CD3 immunostain. (b) Common sites of presentation: widespread small-volume lymph nodes and spleen.

Anaplastic large-cell lymphoma

The T-cell anaplastic large-cell lymphomas can be divided according to whether the tumor is localized to the skin (primary cutaneous T-cell anaplastic lymphoma) or whether the tumor cell expresses anaplastic lymphoma kinase (ALK) (Table 7.4).

Pathology. The malignant cells are characteristically large and express the T-cell marker CD3 together with CD30. They are further divided according to their expression of ALK, which can be demonstrated using routine immunohistochemistry techniques in stained paraffin sections

TABLE 7.4

Characteristics of anaplastic large-cell lymphoma

- Often affects young men (especially in cases positive for anaplastic lymphoma kinase [ALK])
- Extranodal involvement common (e.g. skin, liver, bone, brain)
- ALK-positive subtype responds well to treatment
- ALK-negative disease usually seen in older patients and carries worse prognosis
- Pathology: infiltration by polymorphic T cells, classically with a kidney-shaped nucleus
- Immunophenotype: CD3+, CD4+, CD30+
- Cytogenetics: t(2;5) in ALK-positive disease

(Figure 7.5). ALK expression is due to a fusion gene produced by the t(2;5) translocation. This translocation juxtaposes the genes for ALK and nucleophosmin. The translocation is easily identified using fluorescence in-situ hybridization or reverse transcription polymerase chain reaction.

Clinical presentation. The localized cutaneous anaplastic large-cell tumor does not usually express translocated ALK. The purplish/reddish raised skin lesions typical of the disorder will often undergo spontaneous regression and healing. Radiotherapy may occasionally be used for more stubborn or unsightly lesions.

ALK-positive lymphomas tend to occur in younger patients, produce systemic rather than isolated cutaneous disease, and are generally very chemoresponsive. The tumor may present as lymphadenopathy (which is sometimes surprisingly bulky), bone lesions or occasionally with peripheral blood involvement in which case the prognosis is usually poor. Systemic anaplastic lymphoma that does not express translocated ALK(ALK negative) has a very poor prognosis and the disease often progresses during chemotherapy or relapses soon after the completion of treatment.

(a)

(c)

(b)

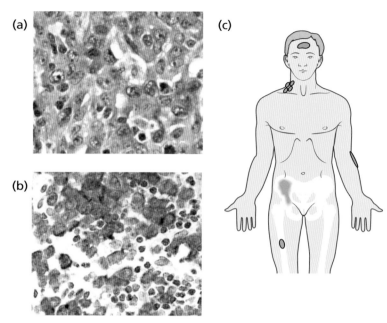

Figure 7.5 Anaplastic large-cell lymphoma. (a) Hematoxylin–eosin stain showing infiltration by anaplastic lymphoid cells. (b) Immunostain for anaplastic lymphoma kinase. (c) Common sites of presentation: at risk of CNS involvement, skin, lymph nodes, bone and bone marrow.

Angio-immunoblastic lymphoma

Angio-immunoblastic lymphoma is a rare T-cell lymphoma that presents with some well-recognized clinical features together with a complicated histological appearance (Table 7.5).

Pathology. The histological appearance varies from 'reactive looking' to frankly and obviously malignant. Lymph-node biopsies show destruction of the normal architecture, particularly ablation of normal B-cell follicles, an infiltrate of malignant T cells that are usually CD4+ and CD10+, and a proliferation of small blood vessels (Figure 7.6). In addition, there may be a proliferation of mature B cells including plasma cells, which presumably generate the high levels of immunoglobulin found in patients with this disorder. A proliferation of dendritic cells is also seen with the appropriate immunostain, though this is not specific

TABLE 7.5

Characteristics of angio-immunoblastic T-cell lymphoma

- Rare disorder that may have an aggressive or relatively indolent clinical course
- Presents with widespread lymphadenopathy, fever, rash, hemolytic anemia, polyclonal hypergammaglobulinemia
- Pathology: T-cell infiltrate with marked vascular proliferation along with a reactive B-cell background
- Immunophenotype: CD3+, CD4+, CD10+/-.

for angio-immunoblastic lymphoma. Recent evidence suggests that the malignant T cell may be derived from the follicular T cell, which would certainly help explain the B-cell stimulation that occurs.

Clinical presentation includes fever, widespread lymphadenopathy, hepatosplenomegaly, hypergammaglobulinemia and, not uncommonly, autoimmune hemolytic anemia. Other autoimmune features, such as arthritis and skin rashes, may also be present.

Treatment. The disease is usually aggressive and the optimal treatment has not been defined. Although combination chemotherapy, such as CHOP, is used frequently, the results are poor and novel treatments are being evaluated. Occasionally, patients may run a more indolent course and respond well to single-agent chemotherapy or corticosteroids.

Enteropathy-type T-cell lymphoma

Enteropathy-type T-cell lymphoma characteristically presents with features of small-bowel disease, such as perforation, obstruction, bleeding or malabsorption. Many patients succumb early in the course of disease because of their poor nutritional state. Several studies have attempted to assess the risk of this disease in patients with celiac disease, but conclusions are difficult to draw because of the rarity of the lymphoma. It is also clear that, in many patients, the enteropathy is diagnosed at the time of lymphoma presentation.

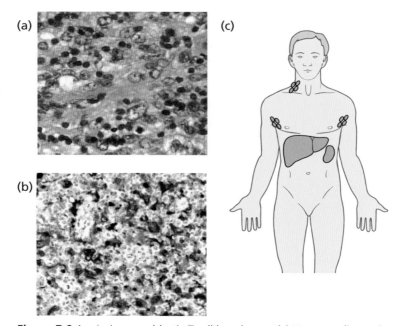

Figure 7.6 Angio-immunoblastic T-cell lymphoma. (a) Hematoxylin–eosin stained section showing prominent proliferation of small blood vessels. (b) Immunostain for S100 showing a proliferation of dendritic cells. (c) Common sites of presentation: lymph nodes (widespread), liver and spleen.

Pathology. The small bowel may be affected by lymphoma, producing multifocal, ulcerative lesions, which arise on a background of subtotal villous atrophy caused by gluten intolerance. Celiac disease is classically associated with an increase in intra-epithelial lymphocytes from which the enteropathy-type T-cell lymphoma arises. Such cells typically express CD3, CD7 and CD103, but are often negative for CD4 and CD8.

Treatment. Initial management may involve surgical resection followed by combination chemotherapy, usually CHOP. Supportive care is crucial for such patients, because of their poor nutritional state. High-dose therapy may confer some benefit in patients who respond to initial therapy and who have a good performance status. However, the outcome is generally considered to be poor.

Natural-killer cell ('nasal') lymphoma

NK lymphomas are extremely aggressive tumors that characteristically arise in the nasal septum and adjacent structures. The tumors are locally destructive and difficult to treat. They appear to be more common in patients from Southeast Asia. Some patients present with systemic involvement, sometimes with circulating malignant cells in the peripheral blood, and skin involvement.

Pathology. The tumor expresses an NK phenotype (CD56+) and is almost always positive for Epstein–Barr virus.

Clinical presentation. Patients present with nasal stuffiness, nasal discharge or more obvious evidence of bony destruction.

Treatment. The tumor is often resistant to both chemotherapy and radiotherapy. Most centers will use radiotherapy as first-line treatment to limit the destruction of facial structures and then use combination chemotherapy to reduce the chance of systemic relapse. Most patients survive for only a few months.

Mycosis fungoides and Sézary syndrome

Mycosis fungoides is the most common cutaneous lymphoma. It is rare in individuals under 50 years of age and typically runs a very indolent course, but the prognosis is poor if the tumor becomes systemic.

Pathology. The skin is infiltrated by CD4+ malignant lymphocytes with nuclei that have characteristic cerebroid morphology.

Clinical presentation. Mycosis fungoides often starts as a single innocent-looking plaque, which is easily ignored by the patient. However, over time, more and more plaques appear, prompting a request for medical assessment. A well-recognized presentation is the 'red man syndrome', which occurs in the variant known as Sézary syndrome. In advanced cases, lymphadenopathy and other signs of systemic involvement appear and carry a predictably poor prognosis.

Treatment. Simple plaque disease can be treated with topical corticosteroids or topical chemotherapy, such as nitrogen mustard. For more generalized skin involvement, phototherapy is the treatment of choice in combination with psoralens. Other agents that may be considered include topical retinoids and interferon; treatment is best directed by dermatologists with a specialist interest in this area.

Key points – T-cell and natural-killer cell lymphomas

- T-cell lymphomas comprise only 5% of cases of non-Hodgkin lymphoma in Western countries.
- T-cell lymphomas often involve the skin.
- Peripheral T-cell lymphomas present with widespread, small-volume lymphadenopathy, but with marked systemic symptoms.
- Most T-cell lymphomas are aggressive and often progress during treatment.

Key references

Falini B. Anaplastic large cell lymphoma: pathological, molecular and clinical features. *Br J Haematol* 2001;114:741–60.

Rizvi MA, Evens AM, Tallman MS et al. T-cell non-Hodgkin lymphoma. *Blood* 2006;107:1255–64.

Post-transplant lymphomas

Epstein–Barr virus. Infection of normal B cells by Epstein–Barr virus (EBV) will lead to a sustained lymphoproliferation unless controlled by CD8+ T cells. Not surprisingly, therefore, when the controlling T cells are suppressed, either by an immunosuppressive agent such as ciclosporin, or some other form of T-cell depletion, there can be a resurgence of EBV-infected B cells. In practice, the malignant potential of such lymphoproliferations (post-transplant lymphoproliferative disorders; PTLDs) is variable; some cases are clinically aggressive, however, and may be thought of as a form of high-grade lymphoma (DLBCL type). The incidence of PTLDs following solid-organ or bone-marrow transplantation depends on the depth of immunosuppression achieved. In renal transplantation, the incidence is thought to be about 2%. In heart and lung transplantation, it is a little higher, but in T-cell-depleted bone-marrow transplants, the incidence has been reported to be as high as 40–60% in some series (Table 8.1).

Pathology. Histopathologically, the appearance of PTLD can vary from almost reactive (polymorphic) to frankly malignant (monomorphic;

TABLE 8.1

Characteristics of post-transplant lymphoproliferative disorders

- Epstein–Barr virus positive lymphomas arise following transplantation in patients on immunosuppressive therapy
- Extranodal presentation is common including central nervous system disease
- Pathology ranges from the less aggressive polymorphic to the more aggressive monomorphic, like diffuse large B-cell lymphoma

Figure 8.1). The tumors are almost always B cell and EBV-positive, though occasional T-cell and some EBV-negative tumors are seen using conventional techniques. The tumor may arise in donor- or recipient-derived B cells, though recipient-derived PTLDs are much more common. As the histological appearance becomes more monomorphic and more like diffuse large B-cell lymphoma (DLBCL), the more aggressive the tumor becomes.

Clinical presentation. The clinical features of PTLD are highly variable. Patients may present with systemic symptoms, such as weight loss, fever or night sweats, or simply with lymphadenopathy. Increasing levels of EBV DNA in the bloodstream often precede overt disease and may be used to monitor subsequent therapy. The common extranodal presentation of this condition means that any organ of the body may be affected including the central nervous system (CNS).

Treatment. Simply reducing the level of immunosuppression may allow sufficient resurgence of normal T cells to control proliferating B cells. (Of course, a reduction in immunosuppression confers a risk to the graft and transplant recipients require careful monitoring.) The success of this approach appears to be more likely in tumors that occur early after transplantation. For more aggressive tumors, single-agent rituximab may be effective, though additional combination chemotherapy is often necessary.

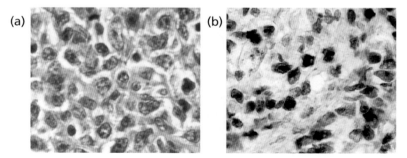

(a) (b)

Figure 8.1 Large-cell, monomorphic post-transplant lymphoproliferative disorder. (a) Hematoxylin–eosin stain showing diffuse infiltration by large, monomorphic cells. (b) Immunostain for Epstein–Barr nuclear antigen-1.

HIV-associated lymphoma

The association of non-Hodgkin lymphoma (NHL) with human immunodeficiency virus (HIV)-1 has been known since 1985. There are several well-recognized ways in which HIV-associated lymphomas present.

- The most common presentation is systemic lymphoma of DLBCL or Burkitt type. Extranodal disease is more common than in HIV-negative patients. As with other forms of HIV-associated lymphoma, EBV positivity is a frequent finding.
- Primary CNS lymphoma may occur in the context of very low CD4 counts. Clearly, with better HIV treatment the incidence of this form of HIV-associated lymphoma is diminishing.
- The rarest HIV-associated lymphoma is the so-called 'body cavity' or primary effusion lymphoma, which is also associated with human herpes virus type 8 (HHV-8) coinfection. These lymphomas are aggressive and present in the late stages of HIV infection causing the accumulation of ascites, and pericardial and pleural effusions.
- Plasmablastic lymphoma occurs almost exclusively in patients with HIV, and presents with lesions affecting the jaw and oral mucosa, though other extranodal sites may be involved. They are CD20 negative, extremely aggressive and the majority of patients will die of their lymphoma despite intensive chemotherapy.

Treatment of HIV-associated lymphoma is directed by its pathological subtype. DLBCL is usually treated with CHOP, whereas Burkitt lymphoma is treated with CODOX-M/IVAC. These patients are at risk of CNS involvement and will receive intrathecal or high-dose methotrexate/cytarabine. All patients should receive highly active antiretroviral therapy (HAART) during chemotherapy. The addition of rituximab is more controversial; some trials have demonstrated a benefit but others have shown an increase in serious infections when rituximab is combined with chemotherapy. The International Prognostic Index applies to HIV-associated lymphomas; in addition, a low CD4 count confers a poorer prognosis.

Treatment of relapsed HIV-associated lymphomas is difficult. These patients frequently do not tolerate high-dose therapy well and its use may therefore be confined to those with better-controlled HIV disease.

Key points – immunocompromised and HIV-positive patients

- Immunosuppression is a major risk factor for the development of B-cell lymphoma.
- Viruses, such as Epstein–Barr virus (associated with post-transplant lymphoproliferative disorder, Burkitt lymphoma and diffuse large B-cell lymphoma) and human herpes virus 8 (associated with primary effusion lymphoma) are often implicated.
- Treatment should target the lymphoma and the cause of the immunosuppression (i.e. highly active antiretroviral therapy in lymphomas associated with HIV and a reduction in therapeutic immunosuppression in post-transplant lymphoproliferative disorder).
- Improved HIV treatment is leading to a falling incidence of HIV-associated lymphoma.
- The use of rituximab in HIV-associated lymphomas is controversial; some data suggest that the infection rate is higher when it is used.

Key references

Behler CM, Kaplan LD. Advances in the management of HIV-related non-Hodgkin lymphoma. *Curr Opin Oncol* 2006;18:437–43.

Kaplan LD, Lee JY, Ambinder RF et al. Rituximab does not improve clinical outcome in a randomized phase 3 trial of CHOP with or without rituximab in patients with HIV-associated non-Hodgkin lymphoma: AIDS-Malignancies Consortium Trial 010. *Blood* 2005;106:1538–43.

LaCasce AS. Post-transplant lymphoproliferative disorders. *Oncologist* 2006;11:674–80.

Hodgkin lymphoma generally affects young people and can be cured in most cases. For many years, the nature of the disease was unclear due to some very unusual features of the malignant cell – the Hodgkin/Reed-Sternberg (HRS) cell. Microdissection techniques allowed the HRS cells to be isolated. Subsequent molecular techniques demonstrated the cells to be derived from a malignant B cell. Hodgkin lymphoma can really therefore be regarded as a B-cell lymphoma. It does deserve its own category of disease, however, as the pathology, clinical course, response to treatment and prognosis are different from all other lymphoma subtypes.

Pathology

Hodgkin lymphoma is subdivided into classical Hodgkin lymphoma (cHL) and nodular lymphocyte-predominant Hodgkin lymphoma (nLPHL).

Classical Hodgkin lymphoma is divided according to the pattern of reactive tissue into nodular sclerosis, mixed cellularity, lymphocyte-rich and lymphocyte-deplete subtypes; nodular sclerosis is by far the most common type. The diagnosis rests on the finding of HRS cells in an appropriate cellular background of inflammatory and other reactive cells. These cells can be identified by a simple hematoxylin–eosin stain and confirmed by immunostaining as they are typically negative for B-cell markers (CD19, CD20, CD79a), but positive for CD15 and CD30 (Figure 9.1). However, most cells in a biopsy from Hodgkin lymphoma are not HRS cells but reactive polyclonal cells such as T cells, eosinophils and macrophages.

The cause of cHL is unknown, although Epstein–Barr virus (EBV; see Figure 1.3, page 15) can be found within the HRS cells in about 40% of cases in the USA and UK. A recent study in Scandinavia showed that glandular fever caused by EBV does increase the risk of subsequently developing EBV-positive cHL; the delay from glandular

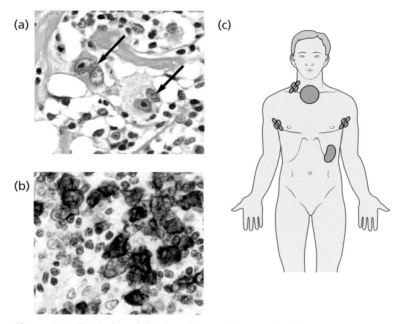

Figure 9.1 Classical Hodgkin lymphoma. (a) Hematoxylin–eosin stain showing prominent Hodgkin/Reed-Sternberg cells (arrowed). (b) Immunostain for CD30. (c) Common sites of presentation: contiguous lymph-node involvement, mediastinal mass and spleen.

fever to the peak in incidence was 4 years. Immunosuppression due to infection with the human immunodeficiency virus (HIV) also increases the risk of developing cHL, though this is by no means as great as the increase in risk of developing a high-grade non-Hodgkin lymphoma.

Nodular lymphocyte-predominant Hodgkin lymphoma is very different from cHL in that the malignant cell is called a lymphocytic and histiocytic (L&H) or 'popcorn' cell. These cells are often surrounded by a rosette of T cells and embedded in a nodule of mainly B cells. L&H cells stain for most of the normal B-cell markers, such as CD20, CD79a and surface immunoglobulin, and are typically negative for CD15 and CD30 (Figure 9.2). In addition, nLPHL has a propensity to transform into diffuse large B-cell lymphoma.

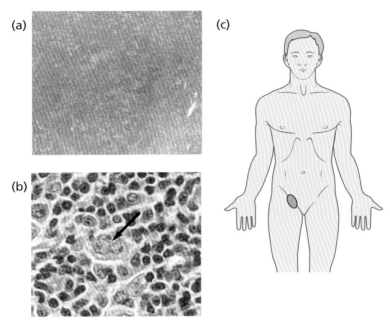

Figure 9.2 Nodular lymphocyte-predominant Hodgkin lymphoma.
(a) Hematoxylin–eosin stain viewed at low power showing the nodular
architecture. (b) Hematoxylin–eosin stain viewed at high power showing
a prominent central lymphocytic and histiocytic cell. (c) Common site of
presentation: early-stage single lymph-node group (common).

Clinical presentation

Classical Hodgkin lymphoma. Around 1400 new cases of Hodgkin
lymphoma are diagnosed every year in the UK and young people aged
15–35 years are usually affected. Like other forms of lymphoma, Hodgkin
lymphoma typically presents with, or with symptoms caused by, enlarged
lymph nodes (Table 9.1). A particularly characteristic presentation is with
enlarged mediastinal lymph nodes resulting in cough and breathlessness,
particularly on lying flat. Superior vena caval obstruction is unusual.
Pruritus is also a common symptom. Interestingly, alcohol-induced pain at
sites of disease is a striking and characteristic feature of cHL, though
somewhat rare. The presence of B symptoms (weight loss, night sweats or
fevers) and bulky disease (> 10 cm in diameter) are generally accepted to
be associated with a poorer prognosis (Table 9.2).

107

TABLE 9.1

Characteristics of classical Hodgkin lymphoma

- Typically affects young people
- Commonly presents with contiguous lymphadenopathy and/or a mediastinal mass; B symptoms and pruritus also common
- High cure rates with combination chemotherapy (with or without radiotherapy)
- Late effects of therapy are an increasing concern (e.g. secondary cancer and heart disease)
- Pathology: Hodgkin/Reed–Sternberg cells in a reactive background
- Immunophenotype: CD15+, CD30+, CD19-, CD20-, CD79a-, CD45-

TABLE 9.2

Adverse prognostic factors in classical Hodgkin lymphoma

- Age > 45 years
- Stage IV disease
- Hemoglobin < 10.5 g/dL
- Lymphocyte count < 0.6×10^9/L or < 8%
- Male sex
- Albumin < 40 g/L
- White blood count > 15×10^9/L

Once the diagnosis has been confirmed, the disease should be staged with computed tomography (see page 47) and occasionally bone-marrow biopsy.

Nodular lymphocyte-predominant Hodgkin lymphoma is much less common than its classical counterpart and behaves very differently. Presentation is nearly always with a single enlarged lymph node and disease is usually at a very early stage. Local treatment measures (such as surgery or radiotherapy) are potentially curative although in recent years it has become clear that late relapses can occur.

Treatment

Treatment of cHL has greatly improved over the last few decades.

Early-stage disease can be considered as stages IA and IIA.

Classical Hodgkin lymphoma. Until relatively recently, early-stage disease was treated with extended-field radiotherapy alone. However, such treatment was associated with a significant relapse rate and serious late toxicities. In particular, it was noted that second cancers could develop within the radiotherapy field. This was especially marked in women who had irradiation involving the breasts and in smokers who had irradiation involving the lungs. The other major long-term toxicity was found to be coronary heart disease in patients who had radiotherapy involving the heart.

Most centers now treat favorable disease with 2–4 cycles of combination chemotherapy (usually ABVD) followed by radiotherapy only to the areas that were directly affected by the disease (involved-field radiotherapy). Trials are ongoing as to whether it is safe to omit the radiotherapy entirely in patients who respond very well to chemotherapy.

Nodular lymphocyte-predominant Hodgkin lymphoma is generally treated differently from cHL, as it is regarded as a low-grade condition. As patients often present with stage I disease, simple lymph-node excision followed by an active surveillance policy may suffice. If indicated, further treatment may include radiotherapy alone or rituximab (as most cases are CD20+), while combination chemotherapy is reserved for more widespread disease or transformation. Although ABVD, which is the standard regimen for cHL, remains widely used for nLPHL, some centers are exploring regimens usually used to treat low-grade non-Hodgkin lymphoma.

Late-stage disease can be considered as stages IIB–IV. Improvements in treatment have led to increased survival (Figure 9.3). Most centers treat late-stage disease with 6–8 cycles of combination chemotherapy, usually

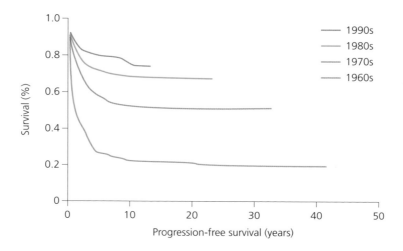

Figure 9.3 Improvements in the treatment of advanced Hodgkin lymphoma have led to increased survival over the last 4 decades.

ABVD, together with radiotherapy to sites of bulky disease. The ABVD regimen is particularly favored because it results in good cure rates, does not usually impair fertility and is not associated with a high rate of second cancers or hematologic disorders.

The main drawback with the ABVD regimen is that the cure rate for disease with a particularly poor prognosis is only 60–65%. Some centers use a more intensive regimen in these cases, such as escalated BEACOPP or the Stanford V regimen. The other major disadvantage is the lung toxicity associated with bleomycin which, if not noticed early, may lead to serious morbidity and sometimes death. If recognized early, however, treatment with corticosteroids is often successful. Vincristine also commonly produces a peripheral neuropathy, though this is seldom debilitating if managed correctly.

The management of residual mediastinal masses, which are common in Hodgkin lymphoma, is discussed on page 52.

Salvage chemotherapy is often offered to patients who relapse. It consists of different chemotherapy agents to those used as first-line therapy. For patients who remain chemosensitive, the standard treatment is to then harvest stem cells and proceed to high-dose chemotherapy with autologous stem-cell rescue. The cure rate in these cases is about 50%.

Prognosis

The cure rate for early-stage disease is generally excellent and approaches 95%. In late-stage disease, the cure rate is 75–80% and, in those with a particularly poor prognosis disease only 60–65%.

As the prognosis for young patients with Hodgkin lymphoma improves, concern is now shifting to the long-term toxicities associated with treatment. As outlined previously, these include second cancers and heart disease. An analysis of survival data from Hodgkin patients over the past few decades shows that, after 10–12 years, patients are more

---

Key points – Hodgkin lymphoma

- Hodgkin lymphoma is a relatively common form of lymphoma that predominantly affects young people and is curable.
- There are two main types with distinct immunophenotypes and clinical pictures: classical Hodgkin lymphoma (cHL) and nodular lymphocyte-predominant Hodgkin lymphoma (nLPHL).
- Diagnosis is by biopsy and identification of Hodgkin/Reed–Sternberg (HRS) cells in cHL, or lymphocytic and histiocytic cells (L&H) in nLPHL. HRS cells are typically CD15+ and CD30+; L&H cells have a characteristic B-cell phenotype.
- Treatment of early-stage cHL involves 2–4 courses of combination chemotherapy (usually ABVD), often with involved-field radiotherapy.
- Treatment of late-stage cHL involves 6–8 courses of combination chemotherapy (usually ABVD).
- The cure rate is 90–95% for early-stage disease and 75–80% for late-stage disease.
- Due to the high cure rates, a major aim of future treatment strategies is to reduce the long-term effects of treatment, such as secondary cancers and heart disease.

likely to die of these late toxicities than from relapse of their lymphoma. More modern chemotherapy regimens are expected to reduce these late effects, but concern remains that a significant proportion of patients with Hodgkin lymphoma may be being over-treated. Although studies often implicate radiotherapy as being particularly associated with late toxicity, the higher-dose chemotherapy regimens (e.g. escalated BEACOPP) may carry a significant risk of myelodysplasia.

There is a great deal of interest in using positron emission tomography scanning to identify those patients who are responding well to treatment and thereby to limit the amount of treatment they receive. This approach would be expected to reduce long-term toxicities associated with therapy.

Key references

Canellos GP, Anderson JR, Propert KJ et al. Chemotherapy of advanced Hodgkin's disease with MOPP, ABVD, or MOPP alternating with ABVD. *N Engl J Med* 1992; 327:1478–84.

Diehl V, Franklin J, Pfreundschuh M et al. Standard and increased-dose BEACOPP chemotherapy compared with COPP-ABVD for advanced Hodgkin's disease. *N Engl J Med* 2003;348:2386–95.

Gospodarowicz MK, Meyer RM. The management of patients with limited-stage classical Hodgkin lymphoma. *Hematology Am Soc Hematol Educ Program* 2006:253–8.

Linch DC, Winfield D, Goldstone AH et al. Dose intensification with autologous bone marrow transplantation in relapsed and resistant Hodgkin's disease: results of a BNLI randomised trial. *Lancet* 1993;341:1051–4.

Yung L, Linch D. Hodgkin's lymphoma. *Lancet* 2003; 361:943–51.

There are four broad treatment modalities for lymphoma:
- chemotherapy
- radiotherapy
- immunotherapy
- high-dose therapy with stem-cell transplantation.

Underpinning each modality is supportive care, which is discussed in Chapter 11, on page 128.

Chemotherapy

Chemotherapy uses drugs to kill or slow the rate of growth of cancer cells. It works by targeting cells that are growing and dividing and that have therefore activated a complex cellular mechanism called the cell cycle (Figure 10.1). Activation of the cell cycle is a characteristic feature of cancer cells and is seen only in a limited number of normal cells in the adult human body.

There is a wide variety of chemotherapy drugs (e.g. fludarabine, vincristine and vinblastine) that target cells in the cell cycle, some of which work in a stage-specific manner.

- Fludarabine is a nucleoside analog. Nucleosides are needed for growth of DNA chains during the synthesis (or S) phase of the cell

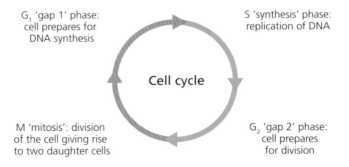

G_1 'gap 1' phase: cell prepares for DNA synthesis

S 'synthesis' phase: replication of DNA

Cell cycle

M 'mitosis': division of the cell giving rise to two daughter cells

G_2 'gap 2' phase: cell prepares for division

Figure 10.1 Schematic diagram of the cell cycle.

113

cycle. When fludarabine is used by the cellular DNA synthesis machinery instead of a naturally occurring nucleoside, it blocks the action of various key components resulting in a halt of further synthesis.

- Vincristine and vinblastine (collectively called the vinca alkaloids) inhibit the action of a cellular structure called the mitotic spindle, which is normally involved in the separation of chromosomes during cell division. These drugs therefore act during the M phase of the cell cycle.

It has been appreciated for some time that using a combination of drugs that act at different points in the cell cycle has a greater overall effect on the cancer cell. This has led to the development of many different combination chemotherapy regimens. For convenience, these regimens are often given a (sometimes) memorable acronym (see page 6).

Side effects. Chemotherapy has a number of general side effects (Table 10.1). Most of these effects can be explained by the action of chemotherapy on the relatively few healthy cells that normally have an active cell cycle. Cells in hair follicles, the gut lining, the testicle and the bone marrow fall into this category. It is important to note that, though these are general side effects of chemotherapy, they occur to differing extents according to the chemotherapy agent, regimen and dose. For example, oral chlorambucil seldom causes significant hair loss

TABLE 10.1

General side effects associated with chemotherapy

- Alopecia
- Mucositis
- Nausea and/or vomiting
- Fatigue
- Diarrhea
- Reduced fertility
- Bone-marrow suppression: anemia, thrombocytopenia, leucopenia

or mucositis, whereas the ABVD regimen does cause hair loss but rarely causes significant suppression of fertility.

The side effect of most concern is bone-marrow suppression, which is often monitored during chemotherapy by performing a full blood count. Although anemia and thrombocytopenia can be treated easily and effectively using blood or platelet transfusions, leucopenia may lead to infections, which can be life threatening and sometimes difficult to treat. For this reason, fever in a patient undergoing chemotherapy is taken very seriously (see page 133–5).

Possibly the most debilitating of all general side effects of chemotherapy is fatigue. Sometimes fatigue is due to an identifiable cause, such as anemia, but usually it appears to be a direct effect of the chemotherapy itself. Fatigue tends to get worse with successive cycles of chemotherapy and may persist for months after the end of treatment, particularly if high doses of intravenous chemotherapy were used. Although fatigue is difficult to treat, many of the other general side effects can be managed effectively with medication (see Chapter 11).

Side effects specific to individual chemotherapy agents. As well as causing general side effects, individual agents are associated with specific complications (Table 10.2). The development of some of these side effects may necessitate changes to treatment. For example, bleomycin-induced pneumonitis is a serious condition and further courses of chemotherapy should not include this agent.

Routes of chemotherapy administration

The main routes by which chemotherapy can be administered are:

- oral
- intravenous
- intrathecal.

Some drugs may only be given by one route; for example, vincristine is given intravenously. Other drugs such as fludarabine may have an oral and an intravenous preparation. Only two drugs are commonly administered intrathecally: methotrexate and cytarabine. Administering certain drugs (e.g. vincristine) intrathecally would rapidly lead to coma and death.

TABLE 10.2

Specific side effects of individual chemotherapy agents

Drug	Side effect	Symptoms
Cyclophosphamide (in high doses)	• Hemorrhagic cystitis	• Blood in the urine (hematuria)
Vincristine and, to a lesser extent, vinblastine	• Peripheral neuropathy	• 'Pins and needles' in the fingers and toes • Constipation with abdominal discomfort
Corticosteroids (e.g. prednisolone, dexamethasone)	• Mood changes, weight gain • Avascular bony necrosis	• Depression or euphoria, occasionally frank psychosis • Hip pain on walking
Doxorubicin and other anthracyclines	• Cardiomyopathy	• Breathlessness particularly orthopnea • Cough • Fatigue
Bleomycin	• Pneumonitis	• Dry cough, fever and breathlessness
Methotrexate	• Hepatotoxicity • Mucositis	• Usually first shows up on a blood test, jaundice in severe cases • Mouth pain, diarrhea – while not specific to methotrexate, can be very severe with high doses
Cisplatin	• Renal tubular dysfunction leading to electrolyte loss (magnesium loss may be severe) • Neuropathy	• May cause profound weakness, nausea, tingling in the fingers and around the mouth • Deafness and peripheral nerve damage

Intravenous chemotherapy is often administered through a peripheral cannula, which needs to be inserted before each dose is given. For intensive chemotherapy regimens, venous access may become problematic, but several devices are available to help overcome this problem.

- A central venous cannula (Hickman® line) is a double or triple lumen line with a tip that is most commonly placed in the superior vena cava (Figure 10.2). A portion of the line is often tunneled under the skin to provide added defense against infection and the external portion comes out usually onto the chest wall.
- A Port-a-Cath® is similar to a central venous cannula, though there is no external portion. Instead, a port is placed subcutaneously and can be accessed by inserting a needle through the skin (Figure 10.3).
- A peripherally inserted central catheter can be placed directly into a peripheral vein in the arm in a similar way to a standard peripheral

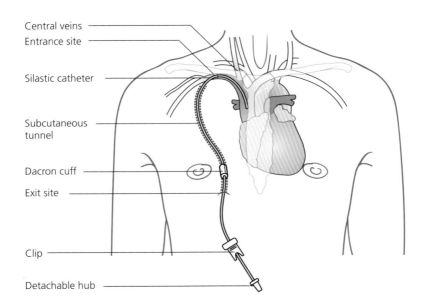

Central veins
Entrance site
Silastic catheter
Subcutaneous tunnel
Dacron cuff
Exit site
Clip
Detachable hub

Figure 10.2 Central venous cannula showing the correct position of the external portion, tunneled section and tip situated in the superior vena cava.

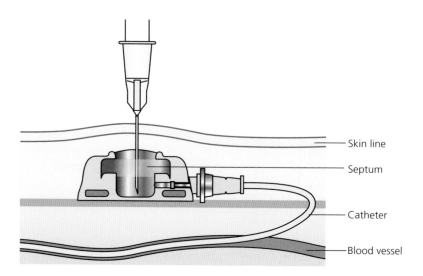

Skin line
Septum
Catheter
Blood vessel

Figure 10.3 Subcutaneous position of a Port-a-Cath® device.

cannula, and the line tip is then threaded into the superior vena cava (Figure 10.4).

Although indwelling lines are convenient for administering intravenous chemotherapy and taking blood samples, they have associated complications. Any indwelling foreign object can act as a source of infection, and a common reason for removal of a line is persistent fever. Also, the tip of the line can act as a focus for the formation of a thrombus. Although it is extremely rare for a thrombus to break off and cause a significant pulmonary embolus, it can cause local complications such as phlebitis or venous congestion in the associated limb. In addition, a peripherally inserted central catheter can cause a superficial phlebitis affecting the arm, but this is usually amenable to treatment with a topical corticosteroid cream.

Intrathecal chemotherapy can be administered in two main ways. The first is to perform a lumbar puncture. Samples of cerebrospinal fluid (CSF) can then be collected and analyzed for the presence of infection or lymphoma, and the chemotherapy agent can be injected into the CSF. This is a very safe procedure, but can cause headache either from

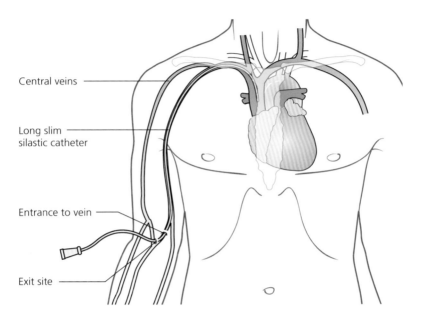

Figure 10.4 Correct placement of a peripherally inserted central catheter.

consequent low CSF pressure or chemical arachnoiditis. The procedure is generally straightforward and well tolerated but, in some patients, congenital anatomic anomalies or previous spinal operations can cause difficulty.

An alternative method of introducing chemotherapy into the CSF is via an Ommaya reservoir. The device, which is inserted in the operating theater, consists of a port placed under the scalp and a catheter that passes through the brain substance into a lateral ventricle. Samples can be taken and chemotherapy administered by inserting a needle through the skin into the port. The reservoir is generally well tolerated and convenient, but infection is a risk. There is also evidence suggesting that the levels of chemotherapy delivered to the brain may be higher using this route and some centers prefer this method to lumbar puncture.

Radiotherapy

Radiation is emission of energy from a given source in the form of electromagnetic waves (e.g. γ rays or X rays) or subatomic particles (e.g. electrons or combinations of protons and neutrons). When these waves or particles come in contact with tissue, their energy is transferred to the constituent atoms and molecules. The main effect of this transfer of energy is to displace electrons thus producing ionized molecules, particularly water, which then damage cellular components. An important result of this damage is to introduce breaks into the double-stranded DNA, which destroys the reproductive capacity of the cell and eventually leads to cell death.

Radiotherapy can be administered in three ways:

- external beam
- brachytherapy (via an implant)
- immunoradiotherapy.

External beam radiotherapy is by far the most common method of administering radiotherapy for lymphomas. To deliver radiotherapy safely, careful planning is essential. The aim is to ensure that the entire target area is included in the radiation field, while normal organs receive as little radiation as possible. To achieve this, several X-ray, computed tomography and magnetic resonance imaging studies are usually carried out. The patient is then put into a simulator, which is almost identical to the radiotherapy machine but does not actually deliver therapy. Information from the scans and from the simulator is then used to calculate the optimum radiation field, and the number and direction of the beams. To ensure that the radiation is delivered to exactly the same place every time, very small tattoos are made on the patient's skin, which act as landmarks for the radiographers.

Early in the development of radiotherapy, it was appreciated that side effects could be minimized and control of the tumor enhanced if the total radiation dose was administered as a series of smaller doses (fractionation) rather than the full dose all at once. Fractionation allows a degree of repair of normal tissues in between doses and results in increased oxygenation of the tumor, which makes it more radiosensitive and maximizes the likelihood of treatment occurring at a favorable time in the cell cycle at some point during the regimen.

Side effects of radiotherapy generally depend on the site being irradiated.

Early side effects (Table 10.3). Hair loss invariably occurs within the radiation field, but is usually temporary. As with chemotherapy, fatigue is often the most troublesome side effect, but it does improve once the course has finished.

Late side effects occur some time after the course of radiotherapy has finished. Perhaps the greatest concern is the risk of a second cancer developing. In women who have had their chest irradiated, breast cancer is the biggest concern and may increase the lifetime risk to 1 in 3. The incidence of lung cancer is increased in both sexes. Irradiation to the neck increases the risk of thyroid cancer and irradiation of the bone marrow can lead to myelodysplasia and leukemia.

Other long-term side effects include fibrosis and therefore dysfunction of affected organs. Head and neck irradiation can lead to a chronically dry mouth due to dysfunctional salivary glands. Lung irradiation can lead to pulmonary fibrosis and irradiation of the bowel can lead to the formation of a stricture. Irradiation of the head can lead to a degree of dementia, which is of particular concern with increasing age, especially if chemotherapy agents that enter the CSF are used concomitantly. Irradiation involving the heart increases the risk of coronary artery disease.

TABLE 10.3

Early side effects of radiotherapy

Site	Side effect
Mouth	• Mucositis
Chest	• Esophagitis
Abdomen	• Nausea • Colitis
Spinal cord	• Myelitis
Skin	• Erythema and soreness
Large areas	• Bone-marrow suppression (anemia, thrombocytopenia, leucopenia)
Pelvis	• Bone-marrow suppression (anemia, thrombocytopenia, leucopenia), reduced fertility

Immunotherapy

A major recent advance in the treatment of lymphoma has been the introduction of monoclonal antibody therapy. The normal function of antibodies is to serve as adaptor molecules, recruiting cells and molecules of the immune system to fight foreign cells, such as bacteria. Antibodies have long been regarded as potentially useful in the treatment of cancer, because they can recognize specific molecules and can bind to specific cells that express these molecules. If cancer-specific molecules could be identified then antibodies could be used to either target treatment to cancer cells, or recruit the power of the immune system to attack such cells. The most commonly used monoclonal antibody in clinical use is rituximab, which binds to a molecule called CD20. CD20 is found on normal B lymphocytes and many types of B cell non-Hodgkin lymphoma (NHL). When rituximab binds to B cell NHL cells, it sensitizes them to chemotherapy and recruits components of the immune system (Figure 10.5).

Rituximab has been shown to be effective in both high- and low-grade B-cell NHL. It also has the advantage of having relatively few side

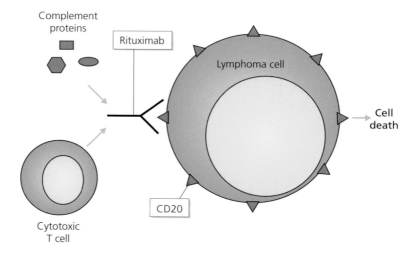

Figure 10.5 Mechanism of action of the monoclonal antibody rituximab. When rituximab binds to CD20, it recruits cytotoxic components of the immune system to kill the lymphoma cell.

effects, with the most problematic being fever and chills during the initial infusion. When rituximab was first introduced, there was concern that the resulting depletion of normal B cells would lead to an increase in the rate of infection, but this has not yet been observed in extensive clinical trials. Certain other monoclonal antibodies in clinical use, such as alemtuzumab (which targets CD52 and depletes both B cells and T cells), cause more profound immunosuppression resulting in an increased rate of infection.

Combined radiotherapy and immunotherapy

A more recent advance is to combine radiotherapy with immuno-therapy. It is possible to attach a radiation-emitting chemical to a monoclonal antibody, thus allowing the antibody to target the energy released. Two such agents are being increasingly used: ibritumomab tiuxetan and iodine-131 tositumomab, which are labeled with ^{90}yttrium (a β emitter) and ^{131}iodine (a β and γ emitter), respectively. A single treatment is normally administered and the most serious side effect is prolonged bone-marrow suppression.

High-dose therapy with stem-cell transplantation

In general, the higher the dose of chemotherapy or radiotherapy, the greater the number of lymphoma cells that is destroyed. However, it is also true that the higher the dose, the worse the side effects. The major dose-limiting side effect is bone-marrow suppression. Although most forms of chemotherapy cause some degree of bone-marrow suppression, this usually lasts for only a few days. With high doses, however, significant anemia, thrombocytopenia and leucopenia can last for weeks or months. The main risk during this time is overwhelming infection with bacteria or fungi. To reduce the duration of marrow failure with high doses of chemotherapy with or without radiotherapy, stem cells can be infused into the bloodstream 1 or 2 days after the completion of treatment. Stem cells previously obtained from the bone marrow (called hematopoietic stem cells) have the ability to return to the bone marrow, grow, divide and produce all the cellular constituents of the blood. Such a procedure can reduce the duration of marrow suppression from months to 7–10 days.

Stem cells can be obtained from two sources.

- The patient's own stem cells can be collected before the high-dose therapy. These cells are frozen in liquid nitrogen and stored until required. This type of stem-cell transplant is called an autologous transplant, or simply an autograft.
- Stem cells can be collected from a donor, who is an immunologic match with the patient. The donor is usually a brother or sister (a sibling has a 1 in 4 chance of being a match), but can be unrelated though this makes the transplant a more high-risk procedure. This type of stem-cell transplant is called an allogeneic transplant, or allograft.

The stem cells can be collected in one of two ways. The most common way is by apheresis. In this procedure, a line is inserted into a large vein from which blood passes into a machine that collects the white cells containing the stem-cell population and then returns the remaining blood to the patient. The procedure lasts several hours and may need to be repeated on more than 1 day. It is generally well tolerated, though a low blood calcium level is a common side effect that can result in tingling of the lips and fingers along with a sensation of cramp.

To increase the yield of stem cells (known as the harvest), two other interventions may be employed. For an autologous transplant, the patient is normally given a cycle of chemotherapy 10–12 days before the harvest. Both patients and donors are then given a course of subcutaneous injections of granulocyte colony-stimulating factor.

The other way of obtaining stem cells, is to collect bone marrow directly from the back of the pelvis. This is done under a general anesthetic in an operating theater, and a postoperative blood transfusion may be required. One advantage of this procedure is that growth factor injections are not required.

Autologous stem-cell transplantation is most frequently used in the treatment of lymphoma. The most common indications (Table 10.4) are relapsed Hodgkin lymphoma and certain types of NHL (i.e. in second or subsequent remissions). Trials are currently assessing whether an autograft is beneficial during the first remission. As the success of an autograft relies on the action of chemotherapy, it is important to determine whether the lymphoma is still chemosensitive. Transplantation in chemoresistant disease is generally unsuccessful.

For the transplant procedure (Figure 10.6), patients first receive high-dose chemotherapy with or without radiotherapy. This is followed 1 or 2 days after the last dose of treatment by infusion of the stem cells in a process similar to a blood transfusion. About 2–4 days after the stem cell infusion, the patient's blood counts drop and an infection often

TABLE 10.4

Indications for high-dose therapy with autologous stem-cell support

Definite
- Relapsed Hodgkin lymphoma
- Relapsed chemosensitive aggressive high-grade lymphoma

Possible
- Low-grade lymphoma in second or subsequent complete remission
- Aggressive T-cell disorders in first remission
- Lymphoblastic lymphoma in first (or subsequent) remission

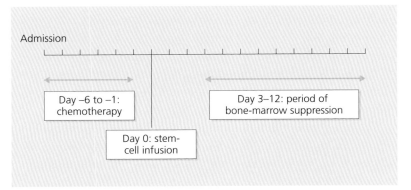

Admission

Day –6 to –1: chemotherapy

Day 0: stem-cell infusion

Day 3–12: period of bone-marrow suppression

Figure 10.6 Typical time line for an autograft. The exact timings for the different periods depend on the patient and the type of autograft procedure.

125

develops. The blood counts normally start to recover 7–10 days later, but full recovery may take weeks or months and the total hospital stay is typically 4–6 weeks.

The side effects of autologous transplantation are generally due to the chemotherapy. However, the stem-cell infusion can produce allergic-type reactions. The incidence of myelodysplasia and leukemia is also increased following an autologous transplant.

Allogeneic stem-cell transplantation. Like autologous transplantation, allogeneic transplantation uses chemotherapy or radiotherapy to kill the lymphoma cells. However, allogeneic stem-cell transplantation also uses the graft-versus-lymphoma effect to attack any residual cells. When stem cells from a donor repopulate the bone marrow of a patient, the immune system formed by the donor marrow has the potential to recognize the patient's body as foreign. When this happens, the immune system starts to attack the patient's body (graft-versus-host disease) and may also attack any residual lymphoma cells. Although this graft-versus-lymphoma effect may result in a reduced relapse rate, this is unfortunately partly offset by the risk of graft-versus-host disease.

Previously, allogeneic stem-cell transplantation always used very high doses of chemotherapy and radiotherapy before infusing the stem cells. This was termed myeloablative, because it destroyed the patient's bone marrow. This led to high mortality (up to 40% in some cases) due to the procedure alone and restricted its use to patients under about 40 years of age. More recently, efforts have been made to reduce the intensity of conditioning treatment and to rely more on the graft-versus-lymphoma effect. These transplants are called reduced intensity conditioning transplants or mini-transplants. This approach has reduced mortality due to the procedure and has widened its use to older patients.

The major risks of an allogeneic transplant are infection and graft-versus-host disease. The risk of infection persists after the blood counts have recovered, partly because the donor immune cells do not initially appear to work as efficiently and partly because most patients receive powerful immunosuppressant drugs for at least the first few months after the transplant. As a result of these complications, patients are often readmitted to hospital in the first few months after the transplant.

Key points – treatment modalities

- The treatment of lymphoma often involves multiple modalities: chemotherapy, radiotherapy, immunotherapy and/or high-dose therapy with stem-cell support.
- Chemotherapy is administered orally, intravenously, subcutaneously or intrathecally.
- Some side effects are common to all chemotherapy agents, such as fatigue, nausea and bone-marrow suppression, but some are agent specific.
- For complex chemotherapy regimens, indwelling venous catheters are often used but they carry the risks of infection and thrombosis.
- Radiotherapy kills cells by causing damage to the DNA.
- Side effects of radiotherapy include damage to local tissues in the radiation field and an increased risk of second cancers. These effects are minimized by using fractions (which also increases efficacy) and by careful planning.
- Monoclonal antibody therapy with rituximab (anti-CD20) has revolutionized the treatment of both high- and low-grade lymphoma, and indications for this agent are likely to expand.
- High-dose therapy with autologous stem-cell support is useful for patients with certain types of relapsed lymphoma and may be indicated as part of first-line therapy for very aggressive lymphomas.
- High-dose therapy with allogeneic stem-cell transplantation is a toxic procedure, but it may result in cure, particularly in cases of low-grade non-Hodgkin lymphoma.

Key reference

Souhami R, Tobias J. *Cancer and its Management*. Oxford: Blackwell Publishing, 2005.

11 Supportive care

Supportive care is a vital component of lymphoma management, and indeed the management of all cancers, because it underpins all other treatment modalities. It can be defined as treatment aimed at alleviating symptoms and complications caused by the underlying cancer (Table 11.1) or its management (see Chapter 10). Good supportive care is multidisciplinary and involves, among others, oncologists, hematologists, specialist nurses, palliative care physicians, primary care physicians, physiotherapists, dietitians, counselors and psychologists; effective communication between everyone involved in patient care is essential. Complementary therapies may also play a role depending on the wishes of the individual patient, and may include aromatherapy, acupuncture, reflexology, massage and homeopathy. This chapter will outline the traditional approaches to the management of some of the more common problems.

Pain

Pain is one of the most feared complications of any cancer, but is uncommon with lymphoma. However, it may occur as a result of:
- infiltration or compression of nerves
- bony destruction
- intestinal obstruction
- infiltration and distension of an organ
- pleural or peritoneal involvement.

It must be borne in mind that pain often cannot be wholly assigned to a single physical cause. Pain is a complex physiological and emotional experience, and not simply a sensation. Anxiety or depression may lower the threshold for physical pain and such psychological problems may also be caused by persistent pain, leading to a vicious circle. In addition, pain may cause social isolation, interfere with social functioning, make work difficult or impossible and lead to difficulties with relationships. A holistic approach to pain management is important, with attention being paid to the doctor–patient or carer–patient relationship.

It is useful to consider pain as nociceptive or neuropathic (Table 11.2). This is not only conceptually useful, but can also guide treatment.

Pain can be managed by treating the cause and by using analgesic drugs (Figure 11.1). Treating lymphoma with chemotherapy may improve pain. Localized pain may also be effectively treated with radiotherapy to the painful area.

TABLE 11.1

Complications due to lymphoma

- Fever
- Fatigue
- Local pain
- Obstruction of blood vessels (e.g. superior vena cava)
- Obstructive jaundice
- Bowel obstruction/perforation
- Itch
- Effusions (fluid in pleural or peritoneal spaces)

TABLE 11.2

A comparison of nociceptive and neuropathic pain

	Nociceptive pain	Neuropathic pain
Cause	Damage to tissues; nervous system intact	Damage to peripheral or central nervous system; other tissues intact
Character	Sharp, stabbing or throbbing pain	Burning pain with or without allodynia (pain caused by a normally non-painful stimulus)
Response to treatment	Opiate responsive	Usually not responsive to opiates

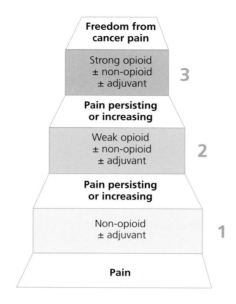

Sample protocol
- **Step 1**: Acetaminophen (paracetamol), 1 g four times daily (if not effective after 24 hours, proceed to step 2)
- **Step 2**: Regular combined acetaminophen and codeine or dihydrocodeine
- **Step 3**: Regular immediate-release morphine (tablets or solution), 5 mg every 4 hours increasing by 30–50% until pain controlled

Figure 11.1 World Health Organization analgesic ladder and a sample protocol.

Adjuvant medications are drugs that do not have analgesia as their prime mechanism of action, but synergize with the effect of analgesics in certain situations. They include corticosteroids, antidepressants, anticonvulsants and antispasmodics.

Nausea and vomiting

Nausea is one of the most debilitating symptoms associated with the treatment of lymphoma with chemotherapy and/or radiotherapy. Factors that must be considered include:
- gastric stasis and intestinal obstruction
- drugs such as chemotherapy, opioids and antibiotics
- hypercalcemia and renal failure
- pain
- raised intracranial pressure (e.g. brain involvement with lymphoma)
- psychological conditions (e.g. anxiety).

Treatment of nausea and vomiting includes both drug and non-drug interventions. Non-drug interventions include simple measures, such as avoiding nausea-inducing stimuli (e.g. smell of a fungating tumor or certain types of food). Avoiding large meals can be helpful, but the patient must be encouraged to snack regularly to maintain calorie intake. Some patients have found an acupuncture wrist band beneficial.

Various classes of drugs have an anti-emetic action and some drugs are particularly useful for certain causes of nausea (Table 11.3). Conversely, some anti-emetics should be avoided in specific clinical situations; for example, metoclopramide stimulates gastric emptying and so should be avoided in intestinal obstruction.

TABLE 11.3

Anti-emetic drugs: indications and side effects

Indication	Side effects
5-hydroxytryptamine-3 antagonists (e.g. granisetron)	
• Chemotherapy-induced nausea • Postoperative nausea	• Usually very well tolerated
Dopamine antagonists (e.g. metoclopramide)	
• Gastric stasis	• Acute dystonias (involuntary contraction of a muscle group)
Phenothiazines (e.g. prochlorperazine)	
• Opioid-induced nausea • Chemotherapy-induced nausea	• Extrapyramidal symptoms (tremor, uncontrollable movements, restlessness)
Other antipsychotics (e.g. haloperidol, levomepromazine)	
• Opioid-induced nausea • Chemotherapy-induced nausea • Metabolic causes	• Extrapyramidal symptoms (tremor, uncontrollable movements, restlessness)
Corticosteroids (e.g. dexamethasone)	
• Raised intracranial pressure • Chemotherapy-induced nausea • Appetite stimulant	• Dyspepsia • Adrenal suppression • Weight gain • Drug-induced diabetes

Fatigue

Persistent tiredness related to lymphoma or its treatment is common and can be debilitating. Studies suggest that medical and nursing personnel consistently underestimate the impact of such symptoms, and the development of treatment strategies for this complication has lagged behind other fields.

As with other clinical problems, it is essential to search for and correct any reversible contributing factors. Potential causes of persistent fatigue include:

- chronic infection
- intractable pain
- chronic hypoxia
- persistent nausea/vomiting
- depression
- anemia
- chemotherapy/radiotherapy.

Perhaps the most common cause is the expected and reversible effect of chemotherapy. Patients should be reassured that this effect will improve at the end of their treatment although it may take weeks or months.

The treatment of cancer-related fatigue involves non-drug and drug treatments. The mainstay of non-drug treatment of fatigue is to create a moderate exercise program. Evidence suggests that this routine is able to improve functional capacity, mood and wellbeing. Other interventions include improving nutritional status and ensuring healthy sleep patterns.

Drug treatments are not universally successful and may have severe side effects. Although corticosteroids may have the rapid and beneficial side effect of appetite stimulation, their use is limited by early side effects, such as fluid retention and myopathy; their effect may also wear off within a few weeks. Progestogens are an alternative with fewer side effects, but have limited efficacy and it may take a few weeks for a beneficial effect to become apparent. Erythropoietin has been shown to be beneficial in anemic patients undergoing chemotherapy (see overleaf).

Bone-marrow suppression

Chemotherapy and radiotherapy preferentially kill cells that are actively cycling, thereby harming hematopoiesis. This may manifest as:

- anemia
- infections
- bleeding.

Anemia is defined as a reduction in the oxygen-carrying capacity of the blood due to a reduction in hemoglobin. The most common cause of anemia in lymphoma patients is bone-marrow suppression caused by chemotherapy and/or radiotherapy. There are two treatment options.

Regular blood transfusions. In many centers, a blood transfusion is given when the hemoglobin level falls below a certain cut-off value. However, there is little evidence to support the use of a cut-off and it may be more appropriate to transfuse only when the patient becomes symptomatic. It must also be borne in mind that red cell transfusions are associated with a small but definite risk of transmission of blood-borne viruses.

Recombinant human erythropoietin (rHuEpo) is administered as a subcutaneous injection and directly stimulates the red cell precursors in the bone marrow. RHuEpo has been shown to reduce red cell requirements and improve quality of life in cancer patients undergoing chemotherapy. Unfortunately, only about 50% of patients respond and it is very difficult to identify non-responders without giving a trial of the drug. There have also been some concerns over a possible link between the use of rHuEpo prophylactically and increased mortality. rHuEpo is also very expensive and not widely available in the UK for this indication.

Infections. Bone-marrow suppression leads to a low white cell count with resulting immunosuppression. Neutrophils have a particular role in the defense against bacteria and fungi, and a lymphoma patient with a low neutrophil count (neutropenia) is particularly susceptible to serious infection. Such an infection is termed neutropenic sepsis and is a medical emergency. Although a normal neutrophil count is $1.5–4.0 \times 10^9/L$, the risk of infection is only increased greatly when the count falls to below 0.5×10^9/L. In this situation, a number of steps should be taken to prevent neutropenic sepsis developing (Table 11.4).

The use of prophylactic antibiotics and injections of growth factor should be considered. The use of prophylactic oral antibiotics was recently the subject of two large randomized trials. These concluded that for both outpatient chemotherapy and high-dose inpatient regimens, prophylactic oral levofloxacin resulted in a reduction in fever and antibiotic use. In addition, in the outpatient setting, fewer hospital admissions were required. However, mortality was unaffected and concerns about the possible emergence of resistant organisms remain.

Prophylactic use of granulocyte colony-stimulating factor (G-CSF) has also been shown to reduce the incidence of fever, the use of antibiotics and the length of hospital stay during chemotherapy regimens associated with a greater than 20% risk of febrile neutropenia.

TABLE 11.4

Measures to prevent neutropenic sepsis

- Monitor core body temperature regularly and seek urgent medical advice if the temperature exceeds 38°C or if the patient feels unwell (hot/cold, shivers, shakes) regardless of temperature

- Take meticulous care of indwelling lines and use an aseptic technique when accessing the line

- Isolate the patient in a side room in hospital; however, the benefit of this intervention is questionable

- Eat a neutropenic diet: products such as unpasteurized milk, blue cheeses, uncooked vegetables, salads, uncooked herbs and spices, raw nuts, and raw or undercooked meat or fish should be avoided

- Employ good dental hygiene including the use of an antiseptic mouth wash such as chlorhexidine

- Ensure regular handwashing by both the patient and those with whom he/she comes into contact

In addition, G-CSF is an integral part of some chemotherapy regimens such as CHOP-14, which could not be administered without growth factor support. G-CSF is administered as a subcutaneous injection either daily (lenograstim, filgrastim) or as a single depot injection (pegfilgrastim).

A neutropenic patient with a fever requires urgent assessment.

- Monitor temperature, blood pressure, pulse and oxygen saturations regularly.
- If the patient is stable, take a short history and perform a physical examination to identify the source of the infection (e.g. line infection, chest infection, urinary tract infection).
- Take blood cultures from any indwelling catheters and from a peripheral vein.
- Request other blood tests as appropriate (e.g. full blood count, creatinine, electrolytes, liver function tests, coagulation screen, arterial blood gases).
- Arrange for other tests that may help localize the source of infection (e.g. urine cultures, stool cultures, chest radiograph).
- Prescribe and administer intravenous antibiotics urgently. These vary according to local policy, but typically include a broad-spectrum β-lactam antibiotic with an aminoglycoside (e.g. piperacillin plus gentamicin). Always check for a history of allergy before administering any medications.
- If the patient becomes hemodynamically unstable (high pulse rate, low blood pressure, falling urine output), administer fluid resuscitation and possibly inotropic support, and obtain advice from the intensive care team.

Occasionally, relatives of a patient with neutropenic sepsis feel guilty that they may be the source of the infection. It is important to reassure them that most infections arise from the patient's own bacterial flora.

Bleeding due to thrombocytopenia may manifest as a nose bleed, gum bleeding or gastrointestinal bleeding. A petechial rash is also common.

Serious bleeding is often prevented by monitoring the platelet count and giving a platelet transfusion when the count falls below a given cut-off value. The normal platelet count is $150–400 \times 10^9$/L, but prophylactic platelet transfusions are seldom given unless the count falls below 20×10^9/L or even 10×10^9/L. In addition, the following steps help to reduce the incidence of bleeding:

- Avoid antiplatelet medication (e.g. aspirin, non-steroidal anti-inflammatory agents such as ibuprofen, diclofenac).
- Avoid intramuscular injections which may result in painful intramuscular hematomas.
- Ensure the platelet count is sufficiently high to cover any planned invasive procedures.

Tumor lysis syndrome

Tumor lysis syndrome is a potentially devastating complication of aggressive lymphomas and their treatment. It can be defined as the metabolic consequence of a rapidly proliferating malignancy and can occur before or, more usually, after the onset of initial treatment. When a cell dies, it results in the release of:

- phosphate
- potassium
- purine nucleotides, which are broken down to uric acid.

Cell death also leads to a decrease in the blood calcium level as it precipitates in the body as a result of the raised phosphate level. The most feared complications of tumor lysis syndrome are abnormal, potentially fatal, cardiac rhythm disturbances due to the high potassium, renal failure due to the deposition of uric acid in the kidneys and convulsions due to abnormal electrolytes. The key to managing tumor lysis syndrome is to recognize patients who are at risk (Table 11.5) and to institute effective preventative measures as follows.

- Vigorous hydration with intravenous fluids should be administered and combined with careful recording of fluid balance.
- For patients at low risk, allopurinol may be given orally; this prevents uric acid production but may increase deposition of other compounds.
- For patients at high risk, intravenous rasburicase (recombinant urate oxidase, which breaks down uric acid into highly soluble products)

TABLE 11.5

Risk factors for tumor lysis syndrome

- Pre-existing kidney impairment or reduced urine output
- Dehydration
- Acidic urine
- High proliferative index of tumor (e.g. Burkitt lymphoma)
- High burden of disease
- High sensitivity of tumor to proposed therapy

should be administered to prevent deposition of uric acid in the kidneys.
- Serum potassium, calcium, phosphate, uric acid and creatinine should be monitored frequently.
- Cardiac monitoring may be appropriate in high-risk cases.

Some centers will administer bicarbonate-containing intravenous fluids to alkalinize the urine, thereby reducing the deposition of uric acid. However, this strategy is controversial as it may increase the deposition of xanthine crystals which can also impair renal function.

Treatment of established tumor lysis syndrome is aimed at treating the effects of the metabolic derangements. If the kidneys fail, dialysis may be needed. If the potassium level is high, intravenous insulin and dextrose may be needed to bring the level down and, if the phosphate level is high, oral aluminum hydroxide may be needed to prevent absorption of more phosphate. Care needs to be taken if calcium levels are low because administering calcium may lead to increased calcium phosphate deposition, which may worsen renal failure. Calcium should therefore only be given if the low level is causing symptoms, such as paresthesias or muscle spasms.

Key points – supportive care

- Supportive care is aimed at managing the complications of treatment for lymphoma or of the lymphoma itself.
- Effective supportive care involves a multidisciplinary and holistic approach with consideration of psychosocial and physical factors.
- Effective analgesia and anti-emesis has revolutionized supportive care, but fatigue remains debilitating, common and hard to manage.
- Bone-marrow suppression is a common complication of lymphoma therapy and results in anemia, a low platelet count with bleeding, and a low white cell count and infection risk.
- Anemia may be treated with recombinant human erythropoietin or blood transfusions.
- If sufficiently severe, a low platelet count may be treated with platelet transfusions.
- The treatment of neutropenic sepsis is a medical emergency and requires prompt assessment by a medical team with rapid administration of broad-spectrum antibiotics.
- Tumor lysis syndrome is a serious complication of aggressive lymphomas. Recognizing patients at high risk and implementing effective preventative measures is the mainstay of treatment.

Key references

Bucaneve G, Micozzi A, Menichetti F et al. Levofloxacin to prevent bacterial infection in patients with cancer and neutropenia. *N Engl J Med* 2005;353:977–87.

Cairo MS, Bishop M. Tumor lysis syndrome: new therapeutic strategies and classification. *Br J Haematol* 2004;127:3–11.

Cullen M, Steven N, Billingham L et al. Antibacterial prophylaxis after chemotherapy for solid tumors and lymphomas. *N Engl J Med* 2005;353:988–98.

Donowitz GR, Maki DG, Crnich CJ et al. Infections in the neutropenic patient – new views of an old problem. *Hematology Am Soc Hematol Educ Program* 2001;113–39.

Smith TJ, Khatcheressian J, Lyman GH et al. 2006 update of recommendations for the use of white blood cell growth factors: an evidence-based clinical practice guideline. *J Clin Oncol* 2006;24:3187–205.

Appendix: classification of lymphoma

B-cell neoplasms

Precursor B-cell neoplasms

Precursor B lymphoblastic leukemia/lymphoma

- Common type of leukemia in children
- Fatal if left untreated; needs multi-agent chemotherapy with CNS prophylaxis to prevent CNS relapse

Peripheral B-cell neoplasms

B-cell chronic lymphocytic leukemia / prolymphocytic leukemia / small lymphocytic lymphoma

- Chronic lymphocytic leukemia is the most common type of leukemia found in adults > 50 years of age
- Presents with lymphocytosis, progresses to lymphadenopathy, hepatosplenomegaly and bone-marrow failure

Immunocytoma – Waldenström macroglobulinemia

- Indolent lymphoma presenting with bone-marrow involvement, lymphadenopathy and hepatosplenomegaly
- Typically associated with immunoglobulin M paraprotein, which may cause hyperviscosity or coagulation problems

Mantle cell lymphoma

- Presents with widespread lymphadenopathy, hepatosplenomegaly, and bone-marrow and extranodal (particularly gastrointestinal) involvement
- Very poor prognosis

Follicular lymphoma

- Indolent lymphoma presenting with lymphadenopathy, bone-marrow involvement and hepatosplenomegaly
- High rate of transformation to large-cell lymphoma

Marginal zone B-cell lymphoma (includes MALT lymphomas and splenic lymphoma)

- Usually extranodal lymphomas
- The most common MALT lymphoma affects the stomach and is often associated with *Helicobacter pylori* infection
- May be widespread

Hairy cell leukemia	• Presents with pancytopenia, circulating hairy cells and splenomegaly • Treatment with chemotherapy leads to sustained remissions
Plasmacytoma/myeloma	• Considered a separate disorder from other lymphomas • Myeloma is a malignant disorder of plasma cells characterized by lytic bone lesions, the presence of a paraprotein and bone-marrow infiltration
Diffuse large B-cell lymphoma	• Aggressive, usually nodal but sometimes involving extranodal sites • Presents with weight loss, fever, sweats and lymphadenopathy • May be curable with multi-agent chemotherapy and antibody therapy
Mediastinal large B-cell lymphoma	• Aggressive thymus-derived lymphoma, more common in young adult women • Presents with superior vena caval obstruction, stridor and respiratory symptoms
Burkitt lymphoma	• Highly aggressive • Extranodal involvement, including CNS, common • Needs sequential multi-agent chemotherapy

CNS, central nervous system; MALT, mucosa-associated lymphoid tissue.

T-cell and natural-killer cell neoplasms

Precursor T-cell neoplasm

Precursor T lymphoblastic leukemia/lymphoma
- Aggressive tumor of the bone marrow with massive blood spill
- Usually presents with symptoms and signs of bone-marrow failure

Peripheral T-cell and NK cell neoplasms

Large granular lymphocyte leukemia
- Rare indolent lymphoma associated with neutropenia

Mycosis fungoides and Sézary syndrome
- Rare lymphomas affecting the skin

Peripheral T-cell lymphoma, unspecified
- Widespread nodal disease associated with pronounced systemic symptoms

Angio-immunoblastic T-cell lymphoma
- Rare aggressive lymphoma associated with fever, lymphadenopathy, skin rashes and Coomb's positive hemolytic anemia

Enteropathy-associated T-cell lymphoma
- Aggressive lymphoma affecting the small bowel
- Associated with adult-onset celiac disease

Adult T-cell lymphoma/leukemia
- HTLV-1-associated lymphoma with high prevalence in Japan, Caribbean and south eastern USA
- Usually very aggressive clinical course, often complicated by hypercalcemia
- In many patients, disease relapses in the CNS

Anaplastic large-cell lymphoma
- Occurs in children and young adults
- Aggressive, but many cases do well with combination chemotherapy

CNS, central nervous system; HTLV-1, human T-cell lymphotropic virus 1.

Useful resources

UK

Leukaemia Research
43 Great Ormond Street
London WC1N 3JJ
Tel: +44 (0)20 7405 0101
info@lrf.org.uk
www.lrf.org.uk

Lymphoma Association
PO Box 386, Aylesbury
Bucks HP20 2GA
Helpline: 08 08 808 5555
information@lymphomas.org.uk
www.lymphomas.org.uk

USA

**The Leukemia & Lymphoma
Society**
1311 Mamaroneck Avenue
White Plains, NY 10605
Toll-free: 1 800 955 4572
www.leukemia.org

Lymphoma Research Foundation
8800 Venice Boulevard, Suite 207
Los Angeles, CA 90034
Helpline: 1 800 500 9976
Tel: +1 310 204 7040
helpline@lymphoma.org
www.lymphoma.org

International

Leukaemia Foundation (Australia)
Level 4, Mincom Central
193 Turbot Street, Brisbane
Qld 4000, Australia
Toll-free: 1 800 620 420
Tel: +61 (0)7 3318 4418
info@leukaemia.org.au
www.leukaemia.org.au

Lymphoma Foundation Canada
16–1375 Southdown Road, No. 236
Mississauga, ON, L5J 2Z1, Canada
Toll-free: 1 866 659 5556
Tel: +1 905 822 5135
info@lymphoma.ca
www.lymphoma.ca

**Lymphoma Support and Research
Association Inc.**
PO Box 392, Burleigh Heads
Qld 4220, Australia
Tel: +61 (0)7 3030 5050
enquiries@lymphoma.org.au
www.lymphoma.org.au

The Leukaemia & Blood Foundation (New Zealand)
PO Box 99–182, Newmarket
Auckland 1149, New Zealand
Toll-free: 0800 15 10 15
Tel: +64 (0)9 638 3556
lbf@leukaemia.org.nz
www.leukaemia.org.nz

The Leukemia & Lymphoma Society (Canada)
804–2 Lansing Square, Toronto
ON M2J 4P8, Canada
Tel: + 1 416 661 9541
www.leukemia-lymphoma.org

Useful websites
Chronic Lymphocytic Leukemia Information Group
www.cllinfogroup.org

Lymphoma Information Network
www.lymphomainfo.net

Lymphoma-net.org
www.lymphoma-net.org

Mantle Cell Lymphoma Consortium
www.mantlecelllymphoma.org

Index